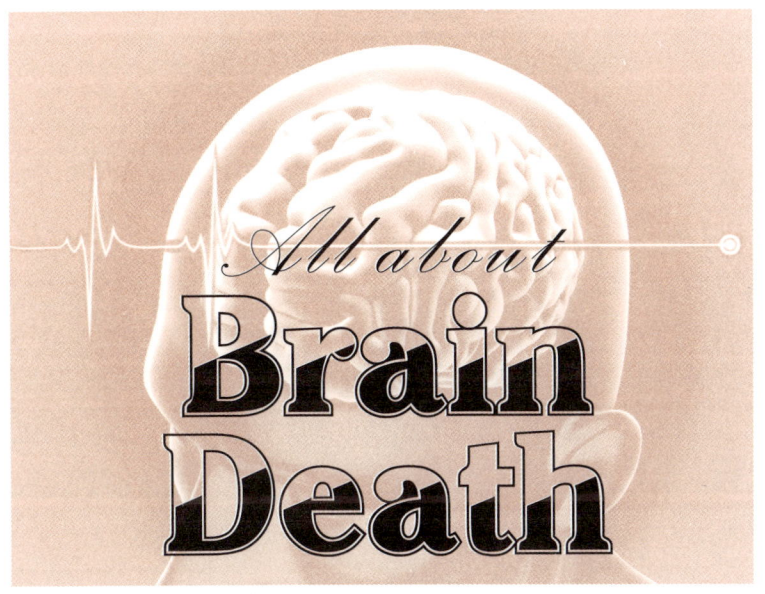

All about

Brain Death

Forewords by

Prof R Arun Kumar
Prof T Kanno

Question–Answer format for clear comprehension

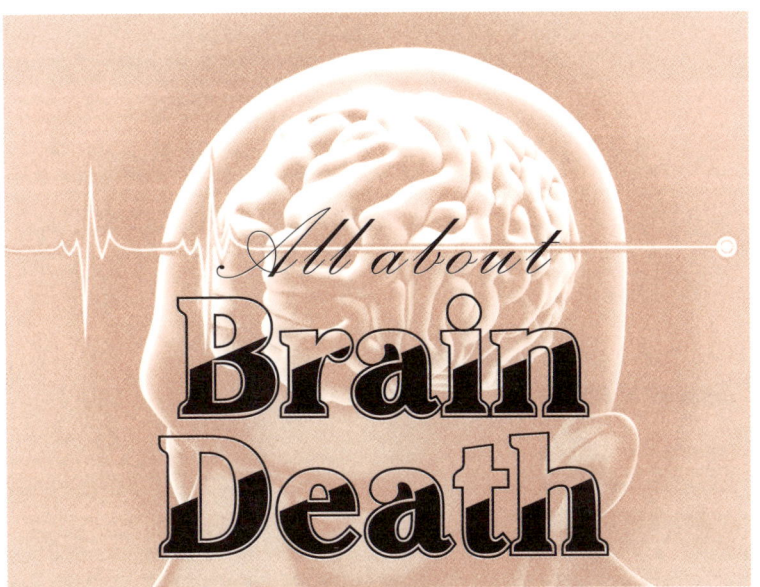

All about

Brain Death

K Gireesh

MD (Gen Med), DM (Neurology), MCh (Neurosurgery)

Ex-Professor
Department of Neurosurgery
Institute of Neurology
Chennai, Tamil Nadu

Neurophysician and Neurosurgeon
Padma Clinic and Nursing Home
Poonamallee High Road
Kilpauk, Chennai
Tamil Nadu

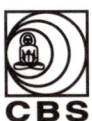

CBS

CBS Publishers & Distributors Pvt Ltd

New Delhi • Bengaluru • Chennai • Kochi • Kolkata • Mumbai
Hyderabad • Nagpur • Patna • Pune • Vijayawada

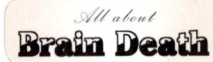

ISBN: 978-93-86310-66-8

Copyright © Author and Publisher

First Edition: 2017

Published by Satish Kumar Jain and produced by Varun Jain for

CBS Publishers & Distributors Pvt Ltd

4819/XI Prahlad Street, 24 Ansari Road, Daryaganj, New Delhi 110 002, India.
Ph: 23289259, 23266861, 23266867   Website: www.cbspd.com
Fax: 011-23243014   e-mail: delhi@cbspd.com; cbspubs@airtelmail.in.
Corporate Office: 204 FIE, Industrial Area, Patparganj, Delhi 110 092
Ph: 4934 4934   Fax: 4934 4935   e-mail: publishing@cbspd.com; publicity@cbspd.com

Branches

- **Bengaluru:** Seema House 2975, 17th Cross, K.R. Road,
  Banasankari 2nd Stage, Bengaluru 560 070, Karnataka
  Ph: +91-80-26771678/79   Fax: +91-80-26771680   e-mail: bangalore@cbspd.com
- **Chennai:** 7, Subbaraya Street, Shenoy Nagar, Chennai 600 030, Tamil Nadu
  Ph: +91-44-26680620, 26681266   Fax: +91-44-42032115   e-mail: chennai@cbspd.com
- **Kochi:** Ashana House, No. 39/1904, AM Thomas Road, Valanjambalam,
  Ernakulam 682 018, Kochi, Kerala
  Ph: +91-484-4059061-65   Fax: +91-484-4059065   e-mail: kochi@cbspd.com
- **Kolkata:** 6/B, Ground Floor, Rameswar Shaw Road, Kolkata-700 014, West Bengal
  Ph: +91-33-22891126, 22891127, 22891128   e-mail: kolkata@cbspd.com
- **Mumbai:** 83-C, Dr E Moses Road, Worli, Mumbai-400018, Maharashtra
  Ph: +91-22-24902340/41   Fax: +91-22-24902342   e-mail: mumbai@cbspd.com

Representatives

- **Hyderabad** 0-9885175004 • **Nagpur**   0-9021734563   • **Patna**   0-9334159340
- **Pune**   0-9623451994 • **Vijayawada** 0-9000660880

Printed at: Rashtriya Printers, Dilshad Garden, Delhi, India

Foreword

For ages, people had considered life to exist as long as an individual was breathing. It was later realized that respiration was the means of maintaining the heart which circulated the blood. Life was then attributed to cardio-respiratory action. As long as such activity maintained the nutritional needs of the brain, the individual was alive. But in the middle of this century, physicians became aware that the brain required much more energy than other organs, and if its needs were not met, it would cease to function, while other parts of the body (requiring less energy) might remain viable and even regain their activity provided the circulation was maintained. The result would be dead brain in a viable body. Is an individual in such a situation *dead* or *alive*? Before answering that question, one has to establish the general principles upon which the diagnosis of a dead brain could be made.

This book elaborates on the important criteria to diagnose brain death in the form of questions and answers which will definitely clear the doubts lingering in the minds of many in the medical profession regarding various aspects of brain death and organ transplantation.

I have immense appreciation for the author, for he has been extremely successful in accomplishing the above important goal and all of us will definitely benefit from this book.

Prof R Arun Kumar
MBBS, MRSH (Lond), MCh (Neurosurgery)
Ex-Professor
Department of Neurosurgery
Institute of Neurology
Madras Medical College

Neurosurgeon
Government General Hospital, Chennai

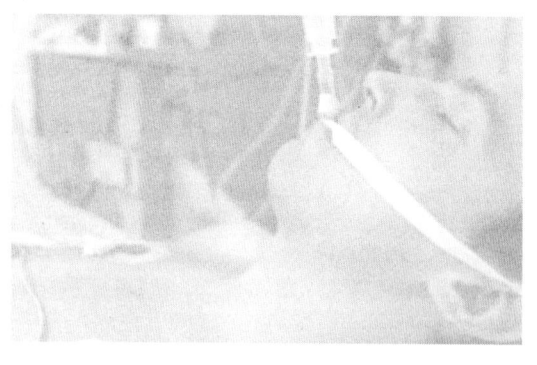

Foreword

There exists only one kind of human death—the irreversible loss of capacity of consciousness combined with irreversible loss of capacity of breathlessness, and hence to sustain a spontaneous beat. All the deaths in this perspective are of brain stem death. A diagnosis of brain stem death has two implications. The first, pragmatic, was that the heart will inevitably stop within a relatively short period. The second, philosophical, was that quite independently of the cardiac prognosis, an individual with a dead brain stem was already dead (because of irreversible unconsciousness and irreversible apnea). In the present volume the author has employed the question and answer approach in describing all aspects of brain death. The book is intended to cover the kind of questions commonly encountered in academic institutions for teaching students, the residents and especially in the intensive care. This book will be of immense use to physicians, neurologists, neurosurgeons and transplantation surgeons of all disciplines. I must congratulate the author for his sincere effort in summarizing the current literature on brain death.

Prof T Kanno
Ex-Professor and Chairman
Department of Neurosurgery
Fujitha Health University
Japan

Preface

Brain death has a history of nearly one full century. In most cases brain death occurs as a sequel to increased intracranial pressure, nearly every neurosurgeon has experienced. In addition, neurologists, emergency care physicians and intensivists may also have had experience in encountering brain death state. The fact is that there are a large number of persons in the medical profession that lack a correct awareness of this condition. This is exactly what prompted me to write this book on brain death. This book consists of answers to questions which arise in anyone's mind when one considers or thinks of brain death. We are sure that this book will be of great use to one and all in the medical profession. The aim of this book is to give every neurosurgeon and neurologist sufficient theoretical knowledge to feel confident in diagnosing brain stem death. There is a certain amount of overlap of answers but we do consider it as a reinforcement of knowledge. A glimpse into the controversies on definition of death and brain death is made. This book also details the human organ transplantation in the Indian scenario.

Further, I strongly feel that it is necessary to educate people to achieve a new culture about the need for organ transplantation. Thereby people would be psychologically prepared when facing the death of a relative to give their consent to donate organs. Indeed organ transplantation allows a dead person to offer life to another.

K Gireesh

Contents

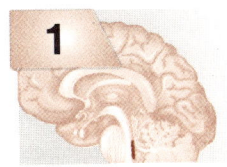

What is Brain Death?

In the report of the President's Commission for the study of ethical problem in medicine and biomedical and behavior results on defining death, death is defined as irreversible cessation of all functions of the entire brain including the brain stem.[167]

Today society accepts that death of the brain is equivalent to death of the person and the death of the brain is equivalent to death of the individual. The physiological "Kernel" of brain death is death of the brain stem since its destruction produces the required permanent apneic coma with cranial nerve areflexia. Thus traditional death is defined as irreversible loss of all fluid flow and air exchange.

The clinical definition of brain death is:
Irreversible apneic coma with cranial nerve areflexia.

The clinical definition of brain stem death is:
Irreversible apneic coma with cranial nerve areflexia.

Thus it is impossible clinically to distinguish the condition brain death from the condition brain stem death. To do this paraclinical methods have to be taken into use, if a distinction is absolutely necessary.

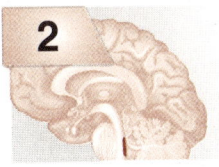

Why Should One Know About Brain Death Criteria?

In the following it will be demonstrated how extremely difficult it can be to establish death in a human being both for laymen and for doctors. At times, it is not easier to establish death as a whole, then the diagnosis of brain death. Here are some examples from literature of the difficulties of determining death.

The famous Flamish anatomist Vesalius was in the 16th century sentenced to death by the court of inquisition, when he by mistake started to make an autopsy of the cadaver of a Danish count, when this cadaver suddenly started to become alive.

To avoid these kinds of mistakes there has been through the years many methods to assure that death actually has occurred. One of these methods was to hold a burning candle close to the body. If the body did not create any blisters, one assumed that the blood circulation had arrested. A dead soldier by the name of Luugi Vittory, who was working for the Pope Plus the IX, was saved by a skeptical doctor, who held a burning candle close to his face. Luggi had suffered an attack of asthma and was afterwards thought to be dead. When he regained his consciousness after the burn by the candle, he could resume his work at the Vatican, but for the rest of his life, he was suffering from the third degree burns on the nose which the suspicious doctor with the candle had given him.

In Munich there is a big Gothic building; where to dead people were brought. A ribbon was attached to one of their fingers after death. At the other end of the ribbon a little bell was hanging in the undertaken office. It turned out that this arrangement was very valuable; because the undertaken was often awaken by the bells.

The most genius arrangement was invented by the Russian count Karnice-Karnice, who was working for the tsar Alexander the III. He invented a coffin from which a tube connected the coffin to a little box located on the surface on the ground. The box could not be opened from the outside, but if there was any sign of life from the inside, the cover of the box would open, and fresh air would come through the tube down into the coffin. When the cover was opened, a flag would simultaneously rise from the box, and this flag would activate a bell and a blinking light to call for attention. The counts plan was to rent out these arrangements in a period of two weeks to persons that had recently been buried.

Even today it is seen, that similar incidents occur, especially at places where there are epidemics and wars. After the war in Vietnam many of the buried American soldiers were moved to the United States. It was then discovered, that some of the soldiers had been buried alive. One would establish this from the contents of their stomach, which contained clothes that they had eaten in their desperate fight with starvation. There was also signs of scratching inside the coffin.

To avoid these mistakes most countries today have specific laws concerning dead bodies and cadavers before burial is permitted. Death is not instant. Death is slowly progressing process, which occurs in different times, totally depending on the special oxygen requirements of the organ. The neurons of the brain are those cells which die first, because of its tremendous oxygen consumption, but electrical activity directly from the cortex of the brain can be measured up to 37 hours after death. Muscle cells after a couple of days. These cells can grow in laboratory for some time. Skin and nails are the last "organs" to die. The growth does not stop until one week after the heart has stopped beating.

During the nineteenth century, these controversies weakened, in parallel with the medical progress (the invention of diagnostic tools as the stethoscope is a case in point), but during the last decades of the same century new controversies and doubts grew up, resulting in a new wave of panic. Here too, the scientific advances were instrumental, the possibility to keep organs alive in the laboratory, outside the organism and later the possibility to culture cells and tissues *in vitro* and to transplant organs from an organism to another blurred the boundaries of death.

Currently three medical considerations make important the application of the concepts of brain death and cerebral death or irreversible coma:

1. Transplant programmes require the donation of healthy peripheral organs for success. The early diagnosis of brain death before the systemic circulation fails allow the salvage of such organs. However, ethical and legal considerations demand that if one is to declare the brain dead, the criteria must be clear and unassailable.
2. Even if there were no transplant programme, the ability of modern medicine to keep brainless bodies going for extended periods with antibiotics, mechanical respirators,

and vasoconstrictor drugs often leads to prolonged, expensive, and futile exercises accompanied by great emotional strains on family and medical staff. Conversely the recuperatrive powers of the brain sometimes can seem astounding to the uninitiated and individual patients who uninformed physicians might give up for hopeless brain damage or dead sometimes make unexpectedly good recoveries. It is even more important to know when to fight for life than to be willing to diagnose death.

3. Critical care facilities are limited and expensive and inevitably plays a drain on other medical resources. Their best use demands that one identify and select patients who are most likely to benefit from intensive techniques, so that these units are not overloaded with individuals who can never recover cerebral function.

3   What are the Important Requisites Before Considering the Possibility of Brain Death?

Before starting the clinical examination there are some unavoidable conditions that must be taken into consideration. These conditions must be fulfilled and confirmed before even considering the possibility of brain death. These three requisites are as follows.

1. The cause of coma must be known and verified, and all possible, but reasonable, treatment of the cause must have been given to the patient.

2. The patient must not have been given any sedative medications for a minimum of 6 hours.

3. The patient must not have shown any signs of spontaneous respiration. A brain dead patient is always on a ventilator.

4 What are the Current Guidelines for the Determination of Brain Death?

1. **The cessation of cerebral function.** This requires clinical evidence of a state of deep coma. The patient must be unreceptive and unresponsive to noxious stimuli. True decerebrate or decorticate posturing is not consistent with the diagnosis of death, although peripheral spinal cord reflexes may persist. The diagnosis of brain death requires that there be no evidence of brain function. The patient must be unresponsive without spontaneous movement or response to pain. The possibility of neuromuscular blockade by pharmacologic agents must be ruled out by history and/or the application of a peripheral nerve stimulator.

2. **The cessation of brain stem function.** This requires the lack of brain stem reflexes, together with the persistence of apnea despite adequate stimulus to breath ($pCO_2 > 60$). If brain stem reflexes cannot be clinically evaluated with certainty, further confirmatory tests are recommended.

3. **Demonstration of irreversibility.** This requires that the cause of coma is established and is sufficient to account for the loss of brain function. The possibility of recovery of any brain function must be excluded. The cause of brain injury can be determined clinically through careful history and physical exam in the case of obvious severe head trauma and/or prolonged cardiac arrest. In general, however, diagnostic imaging studies are used to produce convincing evidence of brain damage, CT, MRI, and in rare cases, cerebral angiography are performed to confirm the cause of brain injury. Metabolic and toxic CNS depression must be excluded. Reversible causes of apparent brain death must be ruled out. These include pharmacologic agents such as barbiturates, benzodiazepines, and neuromuscular blockade, endogenous metabolic disorders such as severe hepatic encephalopathy, hyperosmolar coma, hyponatremia, and

uremia, severe systemic hypotension, with a concomitant decrease in cerebral blood flow, and hypothermia. Loss of thermoregulation is often associated with brain death. Normothermia must be restored prior to the determination of brain death.

Finally, the cessation of all brain function must persist for an appropriate period of observation and/or trial of therapy. In the absence of confirmatory tests, the patient should be observed continuously in an intensive care setting for a period of 12 hours. If anoxic brain damage is suspected, observation for 24 hours is recommended. The absence of cerebral blood flow as measured by radiologic techniques is the only measure of cerebral function that does not require additional clinical observation and laboratory evaluation to confirm the diagnosis of brain death.

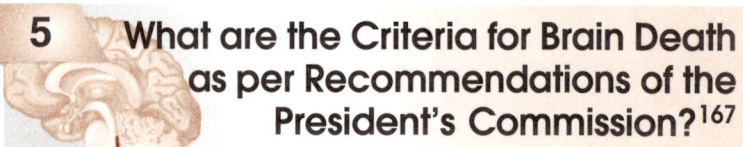

5 What are the Criteria for Brain Death as per Recommendations of the President's Commission?[167]

A. NO EVIDENCE OF BRAIN STEM FUNCTION

1. Ocular Examination

a. Fixed pupils: Absent light reflex (caution after resuscitation see below).

b. Absent corneal reflexes.

c. Absent oculocephalic (doll's eyes) reflex (caution if cervical spine not cleared).

d. Absent oculovestibular reflex (cold water caloric's): Instill 60–100 ml of ice water into one ear (do not do if tympanic membrane perforated) with HOB at 30: Brain death excluded if eyes deviate to side of irrigation, wait >5 minutes before attempting on other side.

e. Apnea test: No spontaneous respiration after disconnection from ventilator (checks function of medulla):

Since elevating $PaCO_2$ increases intracranial pressure which could precipitate herniation and vasomotor instability, this test should be reserved for last and only used when the diagnosis of brain death is reasonably certain.

f. $PaCO_2$ should be >60 mmHg without respiration before apnea can be attributed to brain death (if patient does not breath by this point, they would not breath at a higher $PaCO_2$, not valid with severe chronic obstructive pulmonary disease or congestive heart failure).

g. To prevent hypoxemia during the test (with the danger of cardiac arrhythmia or myocardial infarction):

Precede the test with 15 minutes of ventilation with 100% O_2

- Prior to the test, adjust the ventilator to bring the $PaCO_2$. 40 mmHg (to shorten the test time and thus reduce the risk of hypoxemia).
- During the test, have passive O_2 flow administered at 6 L/min through a No. 14 French tracheal suction catheter (with the side port covered with adhesive tape) passed to the estimated level of the carina.

h. Starting from normocapnea, the average time to reach $PaCO_2$ = 60 mmHg is 6 minutes (classic teaching is that $PaCO_2$ rises 3 mmHg/min, but actually this varies widely with an average 3.7 + 2.3), however, as long as 12 minutes may be necessary, the test is aborted prematurely if:

- The patient breathes: Incompatible with brain death
- Significant hypotension occurs
- If O_2 saturation drops below 80% (on pulse oximeter)
- Significant cardiac arrhythmias occurs

i. If patient does not breathe, send arterial blood gas at regular intervals and at the completion of test regardless of reason for termination: if $PaCO_2$>60 mmHg at any time, then the test is valid (if the patient is stable and arterial blood gases results take only a few minutes, one may continue the apnea challenge while waiting for results in case the $PaCO_2$ is not yet 60).

2. Absent Oropharyngeal Reflex (gag)

B. NO MOTOR RESPONSE TO DEEP CENTRAL PAIN

1. True decerebrate or decorticate posturing or seizures are incompatible with the diagnosis of brain death.

2. Spinal cord mediated reflex movements (including flexor plantar reflexes, flexor withdrawal, muscle stretch reflexes and even abdominal and cremasteric reflexes) can be compatible with brain death, and may occasionally consist of complex movements, including bringing one or both arms up to the face, or sitting up (the Lazarus sign) especially with hypoxemia (thought to be due to spinal cord ischemia stimulating surviving motor neurons in the upper cervical cord), if complex integrated motor movements occur, it is recommended that confirmatory testing be performed prior to pronouncement of brain death.

C. ABSENCE OF COMPLICATING CONDITIONS (THAT COULD STIMULATE BRAIN DEATH ON EXAM)

1. Hypothermia: Core temperature should be >32.2°C (90°F).

2. No evidence of remediable exogenous or endogenous intoxication, including drug or metabolic (barbiturates, benzodiazepines, meprobamate, methaqualone, trichloroethylene, paralytics, hepatic encephalopathy, hyperosmolar coma...); if there is doubt, depending on circumstances, lab tests including drug levels (serum and urine) may be sent.

3. Shock (systolic BP should be >90 mmHg) and anoxia.

4. Immediately post-resuscitation shock, anoxia, and/or atropine may cause fixed and dilated pupils.

5. Patient coming out of pentobarbital coma (wait until level=<10 mg/ml).

6. Confirmation of brain death by use of laboratory diagnostic testing (EEG angiography, cerebral radionuclide angiogram (CRAG), brain stem auditory evoked response, see below), all tests are not required, but may be used as determined by judgement of attending or consulting physician.

D. RECOMMENDED OBSERVATION PERIODS DURING WHICH PATIENT FULFILLS CRITERIA OF CLINICAL BRAIN DEATH BEFORE THE PATIENT MAY BE PRONOUNCED DEATH

1. In situation where overwhelming brain damage from an irreversible condition is well established (e.g. massive intracerebral hemorrhage), some experts will pronounce death following a single valid brain death exam in conjunction with a clinical confirmatory test.
2. If an irreversible condition is well established, and clinical confirmatory tests are used; 6 hours.
3. If an irreversible condition is well established and no clinical confirmatory tests are used; 12 hours.
4. If diagnosis is uncertain and no clinical confirmatory tests; 12–24 hours.
5. If anoxic injury is the cause of brain death; 24 hours (may be shortened if cessation of CBF (cerebral blood flow) is demonstrated.)

Clinical Confirmatory Tests

Cerebral Angiography

Four vessel angiography has been the gold standard for detecting the absence of cerebral blood flow, which is incompatible with brain survival. However, it is costly, time consuming, requires transport of the patient to X-ray department, invasive, and potentially damaging to organs that may be used for donation. Requires a radiologist and technician. It is now seldom used in the diagnosis of brain death. EEG can be done at bedside, requires experienced interpreter. Does not detect brain stem activity, and electrocerebral silence (ECS) does not exclude the possibility of reversible coma. Thus, at least 6 hours observation is recommended in conjunction with ECS. Using ECS as a clinical confirmatory test should be done only in patients without drug intoxication, hypothermia, or shock.

Definition of electrocerebral silence on EEG, no electrical activity $>2\,\mu V$ with the following requirements:

- Recording from scalp or referential electrode pairs >10 cm apart.

- 8 scalp electrodes and ear lobe reference electrodes.
- Inter-electrode resistance <10,000 (or impedance <6,000 but over 100).
- Sensitivity of 2V/mm.
- Time constants 0.3–0.4 sec for part of recording.
- No response to stimuli (pain, noise, light).
- Record >30 minutes.
- Repeat EEG in doubtful cases.
- Qualified technologist and electroencephalographer with intensive care unit (ICU), EEG experience
- Telephone transmission not permissible.

Cerebral Radionuclide Angiogram (CRAG)

This can be performed at the bedside with a general purpose scintillation camera with a low energy collimator. May not detect minimal blood flow to the brain, especially brain stem, therefore 6 hours observation in conjunction with CRAG is recommended unless there is a clear etiology of overwhelming brain injury (e.g massive hemorrhage) and no complicating conditions. Requires an experienced interpreter.

May be useful to confirm clinical brain death in the following settings.

1. Where complicating conditions are present, e.g. hypothermia, drug intoxication (e.g. patients emerging from barbiturate coma), metabolic abnormalities.
2. In patients with severe facial trauma where evaluation of ocular findings may be difficult or confusing.
3. In patients with severe chronic obstructive pulmonary disease or congestive heart failure where apnea testing may not be valid.
4. To shorten the observation period, especially when organ donation is a possibility.

Technique

1. Scintillation camera is positioned for an AP head and neck view.
2. Inject 20–30 mCi of ^{99m}Tc-labeled serum albumin or pertechnetate in a volume of 0.5–1.5 ml into a proximal

IV port, or a central line, followed by a 30 ml normal saline (NS) flush.

3. Perform serial dynamic images at 2 seconds intervals for = 60 seconds.

4. Then, obtain static images with 400,000 counts in AP and then lateral views.

5. If a study needs to be repeated because of a previous non-diagnostic study or a previous exam incompatible with brain death, a period of 12 hours should lapse to allow the isotope to clear from the circulation.

A study confirming brain death demonstrates termination of carotid circulation at the skull base, and lack of uptake in the Anterior Cerebral Artery distributions (there may be delayed or faint visualization of dural venous sinuses even with brain death). Absence of the candelabra effect indicates no blood flow above the base of the brain.

6 How is the Cessation of Brain Stem Function Demonstrated

The absence of brain stem function is demonstrated by the absence of brain stem reflexes and the presence of apnea. Tendon reflexes are often preserved. Tests for brain stem reflexes are as follows:

1. **Pupillary response to light:** The pupils in brain death are classically described as fixed and dilated (5–6 mm in size), without response to light. Factors that may influence pupillary size in critically ill or comatose patients are:

   Small, reactive: Metabolic or sedative drugs. Glutethimide (Doriden) and scopolamine are the only two sedative drugs that cause dilated pupils.

   Unilateral fixed, dilated: Cranial nerve (CN) III palsy (transtentorial herniation with compression of CN III).

   Fixed, mid position: Midbrain pathology

Pinpoint: Pontine pathology vs. opiates (ponto-medullary lesions interrupt sympathetic pathways, leaving CN III, the parasympathetic pathway, intact and unopposed).

2. **Doll's eyes, or oculocephalic reflex, tests midbrain and pontine function.** In a comatose patient with an intact brain stem, the eyes will lag behind when the head is turned suddenly to one side. This lag in eye movement will not be present in brain stem injury. The oculocephalic reflex is never present in conscious patients.

3. **Cold calories, or the oculovestibular reflex:** Also tests pontine function. This reflex generally persists after the oculocephalic reflex has disappeared, so it is important in patients who lack an oculocephalic response. The test is done by introducing iced water into the external auditory canal of one ear. A normal reflex results in nystagmus, with the slow component toward the side of the stimulation and the fast component to the opposite side of stimulation. The brain stem and cortex are responsible for slow and fast movements.

4. **Medullary function.** Lack of medullary function is demonstrated by the absence of the cough and gag reflexes, but the most reliable marker of medullary death is cessation of spontaneous respiration as demonstrated by the performance of an apnea test.

7 Describe the Elicitation of Brain Stem Cranial Nerve Reflexes in a Brain Dead Patient

In a brain dead and brain stem dead patient the following cranial nerve reflexes are absent.

- No ciliary reflexes. No corneal reflexes. No pupillary reflexes. No oculocephalic reflexes (the 4 eye reflexes II, III, IV, V, VI cranial nerves).
- No vestibulocular reflexes (eye–ear reflexes III, IV, VI, VIII cranial nerves).

- No movements of the face on painful stimulation (VII cranial nerve)
- No gag reflex (IX cranial nerve)
- No cough reflex (X cranial nerve)
- No shoulder movements and no tongue movements (XI, XII cranial nerves)

THE CLINICAL EXAMINATION

II. Optic nerve (vision). This can only be electively examined in an awake patient that one can communicate with. Only then it is possible to know if the patient can see. In a comatose patient a bright light should be used, if there is function of the third cranial nerve, the oculomotor nerve, the pupils will contract. The pupillary reflex cannot be elicited in a brain stem dead patient, because light will not be registered, and the third cranial nerve will not be functioning either. In the history of the patient one must have information about blindness or glass eyes and of course, dilating agents including intravenous atropine must not have been used.

III, IV and VI. The oculomotor nerve, the trochlear nerve and the abducens nerve (the cranial nerves to the muscles of the eye). If the eye can register light, the pupils will contract under normal conditions, when these are tested with a bright light. This will not happen in a brain stem dead patient. The pupils are non-reactive to light, because the pupils will not get any impulses from the III, cranial nerve due to absent brain stem function. The pupils should be dilated and fixed, but fixed pupils in a midposition are actually a better sign of failure of the brain stem function.

There must be no ocular movements on head turning (the oculocephalic reflex), in a brain stem dead patient, the eyeballs will lie like immobilized stones in the bulb cavities, in deeply comatose patients the eyeballs will slowly move in the direction to which the head has been turned (Doll's eyes movements).

V. Trigeminal nerve (sensation to the face). If a piece of cotton slightly touches the cornea of a comatose patient, the patient will normally blink. This is the corneal reflex. (Be sure that the patient does not wear contact lenses.) If the eyelashes are slightly touched, the patient will also blink. This is the cilia reflex. These reflexes will be absent in a brain stem dead patient.

VI. Facial nerve (movements of the face). If the face of the patient is stimulated with pain, e.g. massage of the supraobital nerve, there will be face movements of the comatose patient, and may be the patient will even try to withdraw from the pain. In a brain stem dead patient there will be no movements of the face, because of no sensation and no function of the facial nerve.

Since there is no function of the facial nerve, the patient will not have any facial movements on pain stimulus.

VII. The acoustico-vestibular nerve (hearing and balance). There will be no reactions on commands or loud sounds. Before the examination of the nerve, one must be sure that the stimulus can reach the tympanum. The ears have to be examined by otoscopy and cerumen rinsed out. The head shall be elevated 30 degrees and caloric irrigation should be performed with 50 ml of ice-water. Under normal conditions nystagmus will be elicited. But in brain stem dead patients there will be no eye movements. This is a very delicate examination, even in deeply comatose patients nystagmus will appear. In awake patients this is a very unpleasant examination, the patients will be nauseated and dizzy. This is why the examination is rarely or not at all performed in awake patients.

VIII. The glossopharyngeal nerve (sensation to the pharynx). If the pharynx is touched with a cotton stick, the gag reflex will be elicited, this will not be seen in a brain stem dead patient. A patient who is on a ventilator will always have a nasogastric tube for feeding, this tube can be moved up and down to see if this elicitis a gag reflex.

IX. Vagal nerve (the cranial nerve to the upper trachea, vocal cords and cardiac rhythm).

A comatose patient without spontaneous ventilation will always be on a ventilator, which includes that the patient is intubated. Through this tube a suction catheter is passed to secure clean airways. When a suction catheter is passed into the trachea and bronchial tree the patient will normally cough heavily. In brain dead patient there will be cough reflex. By pain stimulus the heart rate will normally increase, but this does not happen in a brain dead patient. The heart rate will be unchanged and low. One mg of atropine can be administered IV to observe if the heart rate is elevated. Atropine has muscarinic blocking effect, whereby it prevents the reflex vagal slowing of the heart. In a brain dead patient atropine has therefore no effect on the heart rate.

X. Accessory nerve (innervate the muscles that elevate the shoulders). Comatose patients might well move their shoulders and lift these on pain stimulus. This does not happen in a brain dead patient.

XI. The hypoglossal nerve (innervates the tongue). This function cannot be examined in presumed brain stem dead patient.

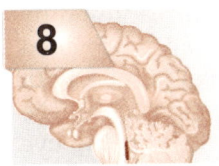

8

What is the Apneic Test and How is it Performed?

A. APNEA TEST (GUIDELINES FOR TESTING)

1. **Prerequisites**. Important changes in vital signs (e.g. marked hypotension, severe cardiac arrhythmias) during the apnea test may be related to lack of adequate precautions, although they may occur spontaneously during increasing acidosis. Therefore, the following prerequisites are suggested: (1) core temperature greater than or equal to 36.5°C (4.5°C higher than the required 32°C for clinical diagnosis of brain death) (2) systolic blood pressure greater than or equal to 90 mmHg (3) euvolemia (option: preferably positive fluid balance in the previous 6 hours) (4) eucapnia (option: arterial pCO_2 greater than or equal to 40 mmHg), and (5) normoxemia (option: arterial pO_2 greater than or equal to 200 mmHg). A pulse oximeter is connected to the patient.

2. **Testing**
   - Disconnect the ventilator.
   - Deliver 100% O_2, 6 L/min. Option: Place a cannula at the level of the carina.

- Look closely for respiratory movements. Respiration is defined as abdominal or chest excursions that produce adequate tidal volumes. If present, respiration can be expected early in the apnea test. When respiratory-like movements occur, they can be expected at the end of the apnea test, when oxygenation may become marginal. When the result is in doubt, a spirometer can be connected to the patient to confirm that tidal volumes are absent.

- Measure arterial pO_2, pCO_2, and pH after approximately 8 minutes and reconnect the ventilator.

- If respiratory movements are absent and arterial pCO_2 is equal to or greater than 60 mmHg (option: 20 mmHg increase in pCO_2 over a baseline normal pCO_2), the apnea test result is positive (i.e. it supports the clinical diagnosis of brain death).

- If, during apnea testing, the systolic blood pressure becomes 90 mmHg, the pulse oximeter indicates marked desaturation, and cardiac arrhythmias occur, immediately draw a sample, connect the ventilator, and analyze arterial blood gas. The apnea test result is positive if arterial pCO_2 is greater than or equal to 60 mmHg or pCO_2 increase is equal to or greater than 20 mmHg above baseline normal pCO_2. The result is indeterminate. In this situation of cardiovascular instability together with uncertainty about the upper limit of pCO_2, at which maximal stimulation of the respiratory center occurs, it is left to the discretion of the physician whether a confirmatory test is needed to finalize the clinical diagnosis of brain death.

- If no respiratory movements are observed, pCO_2 is less than 60 mmHg, and no significant cardiac arrhythmia or hypotension is observed, the test may be repeated with 10 minutes of apnea.

The normal range of carbon dioxide tension in arterial blood $PaCO_2$ is 4-5–6.0 kPa (34–45 mmHg). While that for oxygen, PaO_2 is 10.2–14.9 kPa (77–112 mmHg). When $PaCO_2$ increases above approximately 4.2 kpa (31 mmHg), spontaneous breathing occurs. Without function of the respiratory center in the brain stem, spontaneous ventilation does not occur. The apnea test is carried out as the last examination and starts with normoventilation of the patient. Blood samples are drawn for $PaCO_2$ and $PaCO_2$ estimations and the latter has to be more than 5.5 kPa (more than 41 mmHg) to ensure that the respiratory centre is sufficiently stimulated. The patient is then preoxygenated for 15 minutes with 100% oxygen. The ventilator is disconnected, and an oxygen catheter passed into the endotrachael tube to administer 5 liters of oxygen per minute. The disconnection is maintained for 5 minutes to evaluate whether the spontaneous breathing occurs or not. Repeated blood gas analysis of $PaCO_2$ should exceed 8.0 kPa (60 mmHg) to confirm a non-functioning respiratory centre. Should the $PaCO_2$ analysis be below 8.0 kPa (60 mmHg), the procedure should be repeated with prolonged periods of disconnection from the ventilator.

Guidelines for Apnea Testing

1. Ventilate with 100% O_2 for at least 5 min to produce a normal pCO_2 (37–40 mmHg) and hyperoxia prior to disconnection from the ventilator.
2. After disconnection from mechanical ventilation, maintain 100% O_2 flow to endotracheal tube by T-piece.
3. Continue apnea for 5–10 min or until hypoxia or ventricular arrhythmias result.
4. Follow pCO_2 by arterial blood gas measurements to document a final pCO_2 of >60 mmHg.

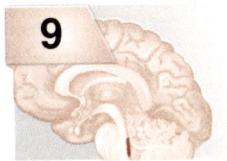

9

Enumerate the Confirmatory Tests for Brain Death

The confirmatory test might be cerebral angiography, EEG, ultrasound, transcranial Doppler, cerebral evoked potentials, radionuclide cerebral imaging or brain biopsy.

10   What is the Role of Transcranial Doppler in Diagnosing Brain Death?

With the transcranial Doppler using 2 mHz pulsed ultrasound it is possible to penetrate the cranium and to identify and measure flow velocities within a defined segment of one of the major intracranial arteries. The blood flow velocity in the middle cerebral artery can for instance measured continuously for several hours with a headband with a receptive socket. Additionally recording of the systolic flow velocity and pulsatile index (systolic flow velocity-diastolic flow velocity divided by mean flow velocity) can be obtained and add information on the ongoing pathophysiological events. The normal flow velocity in the middle cerebral artery is approximately 65 cm/s. In patients with severe head injury the flow velocity is usually initially reduced and later increased towards normal values or above due to cerebral vasoconstriction. A reduction in flow velocity (cm/s) is always an indication of reduced flow volumes (ml). In patient with progressive elevation of the intracranial pressure, the diastolic flow velocity decreases more than the systolic flow velocity and the pulsatile index increases. This happens when the cerebral perfusion pressure (the mean arterial blood pressure minus intracranial pressure) reaches values below 70 mmHg. In brain dead patients there will be no measurable intracranial blood flow velocities.

Disadvantages: Transcranial Doppler velocities can be affected by marked changes in pCO_2, hematocrit, and cardiac output. Transcranial Doppler ultrasonography requires considerable practice and skill.

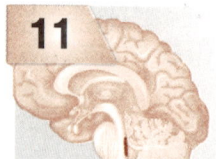

11   Is there a Role for Brain Stem Evoked Potentials (BSEP) in the Diagnosis of Brain Death?

In brain death, the brain stem auditory and short-latency evoked responses are abnormal or absent. The observation that all BSEP components after wave I or II are absent in the brain death but preserved in toxic and metabolic disorders suggests that BSEPs may be useful in evaluating patients in whom coma of toxic etiology is suspected (in particular, barbiturate coma is known to produce an isoelectric EEG).

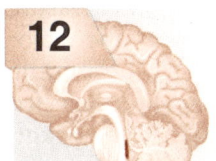

12 What is the Role of Evoked Potential in Diagnosing Brain Death?

Evoked potential studies are used to measure the central nervous system response to signal averaging, it is possible to separate repetitive time-locked evoked potential waveforms from ongoing extraneous physiological activity.

Brain stem auditory evoked potentials consist of a short latency complex of four to five waves recorded from the ipsilateral ear and vertex of the scalp within the first 10 msec of stimulis with a click applied to the recorded ear. Wave I is likely generated by action, potentials in the eighth cranial nerve, wave II is believed to be generated in the region of the cochlear nucleus, and wave III by the superior olive, waves IV and V are likely generated in the upper pons or midbrain.

There have been several reports of the use of evoked potentials in the evaluation of comatose patients and in cases of suspected brain death. Since brain stem auditory evoked potentials are generated primarily by structures below the upper midbrain, dysfunction or lesions involving midbrain and rostral structures do not bring about changes in them. Also they are relatively resistant to toxic or metabolic influences. Indeed, they are usually normal in patients with metabolic coma, and they can remain normal after significant brain stem injury. Thus in some studies of comatose head-injured patients, evoked potentials were found to be of a little prognostic significance, although in other studies they were believed to be more useful in predicting outcome.[91]

Conversely, brain stem auditory evoked potentials have been used as a method to assess brain stem function in patients suspected of suffering brain death. Since anesthetic agents and sedative/hypnotic drugs do not significantly alter their waveforms, they may be useful in the intensive care unit to detect brain stem function of patients who have been heavily sedated or placed in barbiturate coma.

Wave I may be lost because the blood supply of the eighth nerve may arise from the intracranial circulation and thus may be impaired by intracranial pressure rises resulting from brain death. For this reason, wave I should be present at least on one side to demonstrate that the eighth nerve is functional, that a stimulus is being transmitted to the brain stem, and that therefore the test is valid. At least one wave I is seen in 20 to 60 per cent of brain dead patients. However, in some patients, no brain stem auditory evoked potential waveforms are recorded and thus the test is not valid. On the other hand, it is thought that wave II generated in the intracranial extra-medually portions of the eighth nerve, and indeed there have been a few reports of wave II preservation in brain dead patients. Because of these problems, only if there is preservation of wave I and no other waves is the brain stem auditory evoked potential useful in the confirmation of brain death.

Somatosensory evoked potentials are generated by stimulation of a peripheral nerve in the arm or leg. Consistent, well-defined responses may be recorded over the cervical spine and scalp of patients undergoing repetitive median nerve stimulation. Electrodes placed over the cervical spine in patients undergoing median nerve testing demonstrate a small response at about 13 msec. It has been suggested that the generator for this potential is the dorsal column at the cervical meduallry junction. More rostral structures such as the cortex likely give rise to activity 22 msec or more after the stimulus.

Median nerve somatosensory evoked potentials have been used to study patients in coma and in the evaluation of patients with brain death. The bilateral absence of cortical potentials has been associated with a persistent vegetative state and a poor prognosis. On the other hand, early components of median nerve potentials are preserved in almost 70 per cent of brain dead patients. They presumably arise from a generator site in the region of the cervical medullary junction where there is an interface between the intracranial and extracranial blood supply. Despite the increased intracranial circulation that follows cerebral necrosis, this generator remains viable.

Apparent contradictions between tests are explainable. For example, electrocephalographic activity after clinical brain death may indicate survival of a few cells, and the presence of evoked potentials may indicate survival of a few axons. Blood flow may restart after it has ceased if intracranial pressure drops. Conversely, there may be clinical activity when the electro-encephalogram is flat or radionuclide flow study is negative because they do not meet the clinical criteria. Thus confirmatory tests are at times problematic. The results of these investigations shows that to fulfill the clinical criteria of brain death or brain stem death not all intracranial neurons are necessarily without any function, but when the clinical definition is met, no patient has been to survive brain death or brain stem death even with electrophysiological recordable potentials.

In countries where these tests or other additional tests are required to determine the state of brain death, the process of dying is unnecessarily prolonged in the waiting for all parts of the brain to stop functioning well knowing that this has no clinical relevance.

13 What is the Role of the EEG in the Diagnosis of Brain Death?

The EEG is not required to determine brain death. It can be used as a confirmatory test in cases in which the history is questionable and/or the clinical exam is not adequate. However, the following may result in an isoelectric EEG that is indistinguishable from brain death. When one or more of these factors are present, further confirmatory tests that measure cerebral blood flow should be conducted.

Hypothermia produces a transient, reversible electro-cerebral silence (ECS). Therefore, a rectal temperature of at least 32.2°C (90°F) is required prior to the determination of brain death by EEG.

Cardiovascular shock may result in reversible electrocerebral silence. In this case, loss of electrical activity is secondary to the decreased cerebral perfusion pressure resulting from systemic hypotension (cerebral perfusion pressure = mean arterial pressure intracranial pressure). Electrical activity may be restored by increasing systemic blood pressure. Therefore, a systemic blood pressure of at least 80 mmHg is a prerequisite of the diagnosis of brain death by EEG.

Barbiturate coma or toxic levels of other central nervous system (CNS) depressant drugs (methaqualone, diazepam, meprobamate) may also result in ECS, and therefore the possibility of drug overdose must be ruled out by careful history and/or appropriate toxicology screen if the EEG is to reliably diagnose brain death. Most CNS depressant drugs would not produce the clinical criteria necessary for the diagnosis of brain death because of their effect on pupil size (most produce small pupils). Exceptions include scopolamine and glutethimide which produce large pupils.

The EEG criteria for recording include:

A minimum of 8 scalp electrodes, with interelectrode distances of at least 10 cm, and ear reference electrodes interelectrode resistance of 100 to 10,000.

Tested integrity of the recording system by deliberate creation of electrode artifact by manipulation.

Gains increased during most of the recording from 7 to $2\,\mu V/mm$ and inclusion of appropriate calibrations.

The use of 0.3 or 0.4 time constants during part of the recording.

Recording with an electrocardiograph and other monitoring devices such as a pair of electrodes on the dorsum of the right hand to exclude extracerebral potentials.

Test for reactivity to pain, loud noises, or light

Recording by a specially qualified technician for 30 minutes. Repeat record if doubt about electrocerebral silence.

Electroencephalograms transmitted by telephone are not appropriate for the determination of brain death.

Disadvantage: Considerable artifacts in the intensive care unit can limit interpretation.

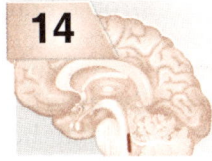

14
What Test is Done to Denote Absence of Conduction from Brain to Spinal Cord?

Absence of brain stem conduction from the brain to the spinal cord is established by the absence of the oculocardiac (bulbovagal) reflexes, i.e. no decrease in the heart rate as a result of eye massage.

Normally massage on the eyebulb will result in a decreased heart rate from, for instance, 120 to 80 per minutes. This is a vasovagal reflex which pass through the vagal nerve. This does not happen in a brain dead patient. The heart rate will be unchanged at 50 to 60 per minute.

15
What Happens to the Spinal Cord Reflexes in a Brain Stem Dead Patient?

A. SPINAL CORD REFLEXES

These may be present, which means that the triceps-biceps-radial reflexes on the upper limbs and the patella and Achiles tendon reflexes on the lower limbs may be present. This is due to the reflex arches for these reflexes are located outside the cranium and have arches for these reflexes are located outside the cranium and have its centres in the spinal cord, which has a normal blood supply and therefore also oxygen supply. It is therefore absurd to include the examination of the deep tendon reflexes in the brain death examination, and it should not be performed. It is only confusing to the staff, the students and the relatives, it they are present.

B. SKIN REFLEXES

The skin reflexes are elicited by striking the arms or legs slightly, this elicits flexion reflexes, which cause the arms to bend and the legs to flex upwards.

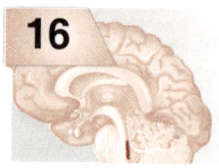

16   Are Spinal Reflexes Absent in Brain Death?

No current guidelines recognize the persistence of spinal reflexes in brain death, approximately 75% of patients with documented brain death exhibit some spinal reflex.

17   What Additional Tests are Available to Confirm Brain Death?

Confirmatory tests of brain death measure blood flow and are more specific than the EEG.

Contrast angiography. This invasive technique requires catheterization of the aorta via the femoral or axillary arteries. A definite test requires the visualization of both the carotid and vertebrobasilar systems. Carotid angiography alone does not visualize the brain stem and posterior fossa, and therefore is inadequate for diagnosing brain death. A positive test is one in which no flow is identified within the cranial vault. Typically, the dye column tapers symmetrically with non-filling of the cervical carotids (pseudo-occlusion) or an abrupt block at the cranial base. This is in marked contrast to the bilateral filling of the external carotid system. The vertebral vessels disappear at the atlanto-occipital junction. Occasionally, the basilar artery can be seen against the clivus. There is no visualization of the venous phase.

Radionuclide cerebral imaging. This is noninvasive, simple, and safe method of measuring cerebral blood flow and may be used in lieu of invasive contrast arteriography. Portable gamma cameras allow bedside exams to be completed in 15 minutes. The test requires IV bolus of sodium pertechnetate technetium 99m (15–21 mci/adult) followed by anterior images recorded every 3 seconds for a total of 60 seconds. Counts attributable to the external carotid system are eliminated by subtraction techniques or a tourniquet placed around the forehead to eliminate scalp flow. With normal cerebral blood flow, sequential images show activity over the common carotid arteries—anterior and middle cerebral arteries—capillaries—sagittal sinus internal jugular bilaterally. Occasionally, the scalp veins drain into the sagittal sinus, resulting in minimal late sagittal sinus activity in the absence of identifiable arterial activity.

   Disadvantage: The posterior cerebral circulation is not visualized.

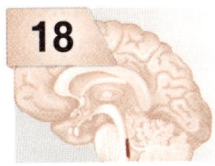

18
What are the Cardiac Manifestations of Brain Death?

Despite aggressive cardiovascular support, patients determined to be brain dead progress to cardiovascular collapse within 1 week. In fact, most die within the first 2 days after the diagnosis of brain death. The EKG changes associated with the initial stage of brain death include widening of the terminal QRS complex (Osborn waves), prolongation of the QT segment, and nonspecific ST changes.

   More advanced stages of brain death are marked by bradycardia, followed by conduction abnormalities, including atrioventricular block and interventicular conduction delays. Atrial fibrillation is relatively common in the terminal stages of brain death, with arterial activity often continuing after the cessation of ventricular complexes.

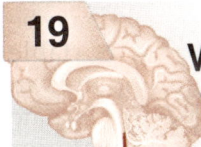

19
What are the Clinical Conditions that can Stimulate Brain Death?

The reason why it is so critically important strictly to follow the basic pre-requisites before even considering to perform the brain stem examination is that there are some conditions, that can resemble brain stem death. These conditions must be excluded before the examination starts. The conditions are:

- Poisoning due to alcohol, drugs, narcotics, neuromuscular blocking agents, sedative drugs and antiepileptic drugs.
- Hypotension below 35°C
- Disturbance in the electrolytes
- Metabolic disorders.

In each of these conditions brain stem reflexes might be absent, there might be no spontaneous respiration and the patients are also in coma, but in these conditions we talk about a reversible coma.

HYPOTHERMIA

The limit accepted when evaluating brain stem death differs from one country to another. The reported range varies from 32.2°C in the USA up to 35°C in the UK. The 35°C limit seems to be more practical and should be used remembering that no clinical study is available yet to define this limit precisely.

Suppression of EEG activity occurs below 24°C and complete loss of EEG signal can be observed with temperature lower than 18°C.

HYPOXIA

Arterial blood gases are obtained before and during apnea testing and pO_2 should be normal. The preoxygenation, continuous oxygen flow and PEEP techniques have to be carried out accordingly.

DRUGS

Alcohol

Blood concentration of ethanol should be less than 45 mmol per L (200 mg per 100 ml). This concentration falls at a rate of 3 mmol per L per h or about 15–20 mmol per L every six hours.[110] Great caution should be taken when assessing drunk patients who have sustained head injuries because they can often combine a severe head injury with a high blood level of ethanol and some degree of hypothermia.

Muscle Relaxants

Adequate neuromuscular conduction can be demonstrated by using a nerve stimulator.

Sedative Drugs

Because of the varying half-lives of such drugs, screening tests and blood levels of identified drugs must be obtained before evaluating brain death. Phenobarbital levels above 25 μg/ml may result in a flat EEG and may compromise neurological examination in infants suspected of brain death even if it was suggested that levels under 60 μg/ml do not cause significant CNS depression in normal newborns.

A blood level of barbiturate of zero is still considered as a necessary condition before diagnosing brain death by forty-three percent of the physicians surveyed by one author.[34]

Narcotics

Opiate effects can be reversed by the administration of naloxone.

Other Drugs

As pointed out by some authors, if any doubt concerning drug intoxication remains, the best safeguard of all is time and the examination should be repeated after a further delay. Urine toxicology screening is recommended if a toxic disorder is suspected.

Hypotension (Systolic blood pressure less than 90 mmHg)

Any co-existent shock with a systolic blood pressure under 90 mmHg may mask potential survival of the brain. The cause of the shock must be identified and blood pressure must be corrected before attempting to perform an evaluation of brain stem death.

Metabolic or Endocrine Disturbances

Serum electrolytes (sodium, potassium, calcium), acid–base balance and glucose must not be profoundly abnormal, otherwise correction must be attempted before clinical evaluation of brain death. Liver and renal function should also be normal to rule out any endogenous depression of the central nervous system.

Doubt

Despite thorough examination and investigations, the referring physician may still feel unhappy with the diagnosis of brain stem death. When in doubt one should not diagnose brain death.

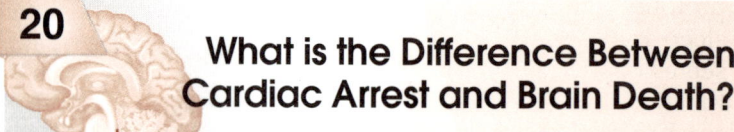

20
What is the Difference Between Cardiac Arrest and Brain Death?

The main difference between cardiac arrest and brain death is that the heart continues to beat in a brain dead patient, but in none of the conditions will there be any blood supply to the brain, and therefore there will be no cerebral blood flow to carry the very important oxygen. But the oxygen will, though, be transported around in the rest of the body and its organs. The kidneys, the liver, the pancreas, the lungs and the heart will not be damaged in a brain dead patient. The damage to any organ starts at the moment of cardiac arrest, which is when the mechanical ventilation, and thereby artificial respiration in a brain dead patient, is stopped. When the brain is dead, the point of no return has been reached. In autopsies it is found that in brain dead patients, where the respiratory and cardiovascular systems have been kept functioning artificially for hours to days, after the blood circulation of the brain has ceased, the brain becomes soft and necrotic and autolysis at body temperature. This is called a respiratory brain. It can be compared with a leg, in which a gangrenous process has started due to lack of sufficient blood supply. Once the gangrenous process has started the leg has to be amputated. A rotten leg cannot function, nor be restored, nor can the brain. It is not possible to live without the brain, which is the organ through which life is conducted, thoughts being thought, and life being expressed.

The brain, the organ through which the soul expresses itself, has been destroyed, has died.

21
What is Persistent Vegetative State?

The persistent vegetative state (PVS) is described as a profound brain damage in living patients, who have regained sleep wake cycles, and yet evidence no awareness of themselves or their environment. These patients have brain stem function, but their cerebral hemispheres mainly in the cortex are diffusely damaged. These patients survive for many years, because the nursing care today is so good. The PVS patients are on examination, awake with eyes open, or they will open their eyes to verbal commands. The patients cannot obey command, and they cannot respond to verbal, visual, or auditory stimulus. They are normally mute and the language is absent. There is no evidence of cognition or awareness of onself or the environment. They do not have sleep-wake cycles. The spontaneous respiration is present and normal. The neuroendocrine function, the blood pressure and the cephalic reflexes are normal. The cerebral metabolic rates of glucose is in a range of patients in coma and pathology examinations show diffuse infarction of the cerebral hemispheres, but no signs of brain stem lesions. Most persons in PVS have severely impaired motor functions with varying degrees of weakness, spasticity and contractures of the limbs, and all are incontinent of urine and stools.

Persistent vegetative state is at times used synonymous with coma vigil, the apallic syndrome, neocortical death and total dementia.

If a persistent vegetative state has persisted for more than 6 months, there is no evidence that the patient will ever improve. It is still widely discussed, if nutrition should be withheld from these patients under request of the relatives, or if the patient has made a living will stating that no treatment will be appreciated in case of persistent vegetative state.

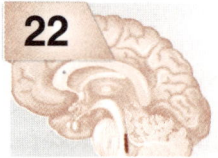

22
What is Locked-in Syndrome?

As the persistent vegetative state is defined as a patient with wakefulness or cognition, the patient in the locked-in state is awake and have cognitive responses to stimuli. But the patients are totally without any motor pattern activity, sometimes also needing mechanical ventilation. The patients cannot talk, the only means of communicating is eye blinking and at times only with vertical eye movements as the cranial nerve functions are also affected. This condition may be due to trauma or subherniation from supratentorial lesions. The condition can also be the result of a lumbar puncture performed in a patient with raised intracranial pressure. This is one of the reasons why one must be extremely useful in performing a lumbar puncture without insuring that there is no papilledema or other signs of raised intracranial pressure.

23
What is the Anatomical and Clinical Definitions of the Following?

1. Death
2. Brain Death
3. Brain stem death
4. Persistent vegetative state
5. Locked-in syndrome.

1. DEATH

Anatomical definition: Irreversible cessation of all heart, brain, and lung functions.

Clinical definition: No exchange of bodily fluids and air.

2. BRAIN DEATH

Synonyms of brain death are: Whole brain death, coma depasse.

Anatomical definition: Irreversible cessation of all brain functions.

Clinical definition: Irreversible apneic-coma with absent brain stem reflexes.

3. BRAIN STEM DEATH

Anatomical definition: Irreversible cessation of all brain stem functions.

Clinical definition: Irreversible apneic-coma with absent brain stem reflexes.

4. PERSISTENT VEGETATIVE STATE

Synonyms for it is: Cerebral death, neocortical death, Apallic syndrome, coma vigil, total dementia, akinetic mutism.

Anatomical definition: Totally or partially irreversible function of the cerebral hemispheres normal or almost normal working brain stem.

Clinical definition: Patient with awake-sleep cycle, no cognition, no verbal communication, no localizing motor responses, but preserved autonomic and vegetative functions.

5. LOCKED IN SYNDROME

Anatomical definition: Irreversible lesion of the ventral part of pons.

Clinical definition: Total awareness with selective supra-nuclear motor differentiation, which produces total paralysis of all 4 limbs and the lower cranial nerves. Vertical eye-movements may be all that remain in these patients.

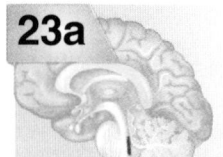

23a

Differences in Coma and Brain Death

S. No.	Topics	Coma	Brain death
1.	Definition	Coma is defined as a state of unconsciousness from which the individual cannot be awakened, in which the individual responds minimally or not at all to stimuli, and initiates no voluntary activities. Coma is similar to deep sleep, except that no amount of external stimuli can prompt the brain to become awake and alert. However, the person is alive and recovery is possible.	Brain death means there is "irreversible cessation of all functions of the brain, including the brain stem". A patient determined to be brain dead is legally and clinically dead.
2.	Glasgow Coma Scale	Composite score of 3, considered the patients are in coma	Brain death patients are usually scored less than 3.
3.	Brain function	A persistent vegetative state means the person has lost higher brain functions, but their undamaged brain stem still allows essential functions like heart rate and respiration to continue. A person in a vegetative state is alive and may recover to some degree, given time.	In brain death, the entire brain has died, both the upper parts of the brain and the lower parts of the brain (brain stem). The brain stem or lower brain is responsible for the vegetative functions such as breathing or sleeping and waking up (sleep—wake cycles)
4.	Confirmatory tests	Eye examination, lab tests, EEG, CT and MRI tests and physical examination, motor examination	EEG, cerebral blood flow study, cerebral angiography, MRI, transcranial Doppler, apnea tests

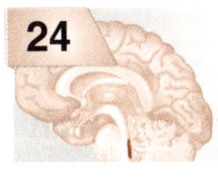

24

Are Brain Death Criteria for Adults Applicable to Children?

Brain death in neonates and premature has always been a subject for debate due to the fact that children can sustain a longer time of hypoxia than adults before irreversible brain damage arises. Also the time interval between the initial onset of brain death and cardiac arrest might be quite prolonged.

This, of course, is only if nutrition and treatment with the mechanical ventilator is continued.

In 1987 an ad hoc Task Force Committee "Guidelines for the determination of brain death in children" was published due to the difficulties in determining the diagnosis of brain stem death in children.[201] The committee, that wrote the report, did not make any recommendations for children less than 7 days of age, because the members of the committee felt that the diagnosis of brain death was extremely difficult to assess in this age group. The reason why it is so difficult to establish brain death in children younger than 7 days is that the neurological examination is difficult to perform due to the normal development pattern for certain reflexes in especially neonates and premature. The pupillary light reflex might be absent before the 30th week of gestation, where the pupils are quite miotic. The oculocephalic response is difficult to elicit before 32 weeks, and the caloric stimulation is extremely difficult to perform. Also in adults who have sustained a severe head injury, it certainly can be difficult if not impossible, to examine all the cranial and nerve functions. If the eyes are destroyed at the accident, one cannot examine the optic nerve and the oculomotor nerve, nor can the oculocephalic, oculo-vestibular, oculobulbar or ciliospinal reflexes be tested. In spite of this, there is no doubt that with the result of the remaining brain stem function tests, when a patient is brain stem dead, the ventilation can be discontinued.

In adults that fulfill the clinical brain death criteria, there can be ongoing preserved cerebral arterial circulation in the hemispheres, demonstrated by angiography, and the CSF might also be pulsating in an intraventricularly placed catheter. One author has in 1993 noted, that several investigators have reported about electrocerebral silence in newborns and infants declared clinically brain dead, but with persistent CBF. One author gives a report of a 2-month-old infant that on the neurological examination, including the apnea test, demonstrated cessation of all brain and spinal cord functions two days after unexplained cardiac arrest (due to head injury verified by CT scan) and resuscitation. At this time EEG showed burst suppression pattern and CBF measurements revealed normal radiotracer uptake. On the eleventh day a quantitative PET scan revealed a significant glucose metabolism in the cerebral cortex and basal ganglia, but hypometabolism in the posterior fossa. Transcranial Doppler ultrasonography showed a high pulsatility index, but the EEG was now isoelectric. Three days later, the ventilation was discontinued. They conclude, that the presence of CBF and glucose metabolism in children with clinical brain death should not alter the conclusion of this diagnosis.

It is thus seen that in children, who are clinically brain stem dead, again follow the same pattern as for the adult brain stem dead patient.

The question is thus, can the criteiria of brain death, that presently is being used for adults, also be used for children including the apnea test with the same thresholds.

In children where the preconditions for performing the brain death test have been fulfilled, the clinical definition of whole brain death and brain stem death is:

"Irreversible apneic coma with the absence of all brain stem reflexes."

This is not any different from the definition in adults.

In countries where no confirmatory paraclinical tests are required one or two clinical examinations, with a shorter or longer interval of time, is sufficient to declare a patient brain stem dead. In countries where paraclinical confirmatory tests are required, such as a cerebral 4-vessel angiography, EEG, ultrasound, isotope scan, Doppler, cine-MRI, etc., brain death is used as the criteria of death and not brain stem death. In children some of these tests are difficult or not possible to perform, as for instance, a 4-vessel angiography in a newborn. If a confirmatory test is desired, then the cranial ultrasound is the best to guide the examining physician.

No one has ever, to my knowledge, reported of a child, fulfilling the clinical criteria for brain stem death, that has returned from the strict and well-defined condition. Only reports of children being sufficiently examined has stated that children had returned to consciousness from being called brain dead. The conclusion is thus, that the only difference between children and adults in determining brain death, is the period of time from the initial onset of brain death to declaring the child brain dead. Otherwise, the exact same preconditions as well as clinical and paraclinical examinations can be taken into practice under the given circumstances.

In the literature this period of time is 30 minutes for children. For adults it is shorter, less than 10 minutes. For this reason, it should not be necessary to change the observation time for declaring a child brain dead from the rules for the adult of the particular countries, if the condition brain death has persisted for more than 30 minutes from the onset. In most countries 6 hours are demanded for the adult.

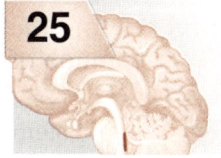

25

What are the Criteria for Brain Death in Children?

Criteria for death: Irreversible loss of cardiopulmonary or entire brain function (as in adult), but the (clinically unproven) assumption that a child's brain is more resilient results in more difficult determination of brain death. The following guidelines are proposed for patients <5 years age.

- In newborns born at or after term (>38 wks), the following criteria are applicable 7 days after the neurologic insult
- These recommendations are not applicable for the premature infant.

- Determination of proximate cause of coma should be made to ensure absence of remediable conditions; especially toxic and metabolic disorders, sedatives, paralytics, hypothermia, hypotension (for age), and surgically treatable conditions criteria:

A. Coma and apnea must coexist; including complete loss of consciousness, vocalization and volitional activity.

B. Absence of brain stem function
   1. Midposition or fully dilated pupils, unresponsive to light (R/O drug effects).
   2. Extra ocular movement; absence of spontaneous, doll's eyes and caloric movements of eyes.
   3. Absence of bulbar musculature movement; including oropharyngeal and facial muscles, absence of cornea, gag, cough, suck, and rooting reflex.
   4. Absence of respiratory movement (usually tested after other criteria met).
   5. Flaccid tone and absence of spontaneous or induced movements (spinal myoclonus and spinal cord movements, e.g. reflex withdrawal are not included).
   6. Examination results should remain consistent with brain death throughout observation period.

Observation Periods According to Age

A. Age 7 days 2 months; 2 examinations and 2 EEGs 48 hr apart (repeat exam unnecessary if cerebral radionuclide angiogram (CRAG) fails to visualize cerebral arteries).

B. Age 2–12 months; 2 examinations and 2 EEGs 24 hr apart (repeat exam unnecessary if CRAG negative).

C. Age >12 months; if irreversible condition exists, laboratory testing is not necessary, and 12 hr observation sufficient (unclear conditions, especially hypoxic-ischemic encephalopathy, are difficult to assess, and 24 hr, observation is suggested unless electrocerebral silence on EEG or a negative CRAG confirm diagnosis).

Confirmatory Tests

A. EEG, standard requirement for 10 cm electrode distance may be decreased in proportion to size to head.

B. CRAG applicability to patient <2 months ago unproven.
Important guidelines after Task Force on Brain Death in Children.[67]

I. HISTORY

A. Proximate cause.
B. Rule out remediable or reversible conditions (toxic and metabolic disorders, sedative-hypnotic drugs, paralytic agents, hypothermia, hypotension, surgically remediable conditions).

II. PHYSICAL EXAMINATION

A. Coma and apnea must coexist. The patient must exhibit complete loss of consciousness, vocalization activity.
B. Absence of brain stem function as defined:
   • Midposition or fully dilated pupils that do not respond to light. Drugs may influence and invalidate pupillary assessment.
   • Absence of spontaneous eye movements, those induced by oculocephalic and caloric (oculovestibular) testing.
   • Absence of movement of bulbar musculature including facial and oropharyngeal muscles. The corneal, gag, cough sucking, and rooting reflexes are absent.
   • Respiratory movements are absent with the patient on the respirator. Apnea testing using standardized methods can be performed but is done after other criteria are met.
C. The patient must not be significantly hypothermic or hypotensive for age.
D. Flaccid tone and absence of spontaneous or induced movements, excluding spinal cord events such as reflex withdrawal or spinal myoclonus, should exist.
E. The examination should remain consistent with brain death throughout the observation and testing period.

III. OBSERVATION PERIODS ACCORDING TO AGE

The recommended observation period depends on the age of the patient and the laboratory tests utilized—7 days to

2 months. Two examinations and electroencephalograms (EEGs) separated by at least 48 hours. 2 months to 1 year. Two examinations and EEGs are not necessary if a concomitant radionuclide flow study demonstrates no visualization of cerebral arteries.

Over 1 year: When an irreversible cause exists, laboratory testing is not required but an observation period of at least 12 hours is recommended. There are conditions, particularly hypoxic ischemic encephalopathy, in which it is difficult to assess the extent and reversibility of brain damage. This is particularly true if the first examination is performed soon after the acute event. Therefore, in this situation, a more prolonged period of at least 24 hours of observation is recommended. The observation period may be reduced in the EEG demonstrates electrocerebral silence or the isotope flow study does not visualize cerebral arteries.

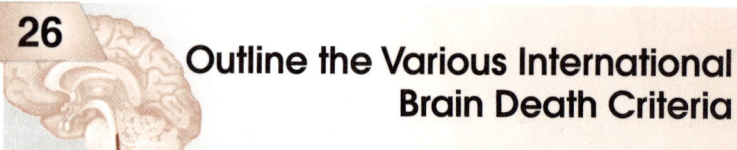

26 Outline the Various International Brain Death Criteria

The diagnosis of brain death in different countries is as follows.

USA

The first guidelines for diagnosis of brain death was published in journal of American Medical Association in 1968. It was called the Harvard Criteria for the diagnosis of brain death and it was made by an Ad Hoc Committee of the Harvard Medical School. The article was called a definition of irreversible coma.

THE HARVARD CRITERIA (USA)

1. Unresponsive coma
2. No movements (observed for 1 hour)

3. Apnea (3 minutes of respirator)
4. Absence of elicitable reflexes.
5. Isoelectric EEG "of great confirmatory value" (at 5 microvolt per mm).
6. Absence of drug intoxication or hypothermia. All of the above tests shall be repeated at least 24 hours later with no change (1968).

Minnesota Criteria

1. Known, but irreparable intracranial lesion.
2. No spontaneous movement.
3. Apnea (4 minutes).
4. Absent brain stem reflexes including absence "Doll's heads phenomenon" Absent cilio spinal reflex and absent tonic neck reflexes.
5. All findings unchanged for at least 12 hours.

EEG not mandatory.

More recently, the American Academy of Neurology conducted an evidence-based review and suggested practice measures, which are as follows.[68]

The clinical neurologic examination remains the standard for the determination of brain death and has been adopted by most countries. The clinical examination of patients who are presumed to be brain dead must be performed with precision.

The most controversial issue related to the determination of brain death is the occurrence of clinical signs that suggest some retention of brain function. Even in the absence of motor responses, spontaneous body movements may be observed during the apnea test, while the body is being prepared for transport, at the time of an abdominal incision for the retrieval of organs, or in synchrony with the respirations produced by the mechanical ventilator. These body movements are generated by the spine, and the evidence of brain death in such cases comes from a consistent clinical documentation of brain death and confirmation by isoelectric electroencephalography or cerebral angiography. These slow body movements may even include a brief attempt of the body to flex at the waist, making it seem to rise. The arms may be raised independently or

Table 1: Clinical criteria for brain death in adults and children[68]

Coma
- Absence of motor responses
- Absence of pupillary responses to light and pupils at mid-position with respect to dilatation (4–6 mm)
- Absence of corneal reflexes
- Absence of caloric responses
- Absence of gag reflex
- Absence of coughing in response to tracheal suctioning
- Absence of respiratory drive at a $PaCO_2$ that is 60 mmHg or 20 mmHg above normal base-line values

Interval between two evaluations, according to patient's age
- Term to 2 mo old, 48 hr
- >2 mo to 1yr old, 24 hr
- >1 yr to <18 yr old, 12 hr
- ≥ 18 yr old, interval optional

Confirmatory tests
- Term to 2 mo old, 2 confirmatory tests
- >2 mo to 1yr old, 1 confirmatory test
- >1yr to <18 yr old, optional
- ≥ 18 yr old, optional

together. Forceful flexion of the neck or rotation of the body may initiate these movements. Legs seldom move spontaneously although in two patients, "stepping movements" (an exaggerated triple flexion) were noted just before brain death. Other manifestations that have been reported are a slow turning of the head to one side, an undulating toe sign (snapping the big toe leads to an undulating movement of the toes), facial twitching, a persistent Babinski reflex, and tendon, abdominal, and cremasteric reflexes.

Confirmatory tests (Table 2) are optional in adults but recommended in children younger than one year old. In several European, Central and South American, and Asian countries, confirmatory testing is required by law. Certain countries, (e.g. Sweden) require only cerebral angiography. In the United States, the choice of tests is left to the discretion of the physician, but bedside tests seem to be preferred.

Table 2: Confirmatory testing for a determination of brain death

Cerebral angiography

- The contrast medium should be injected under high pressure in both anterior and posterior circulation.
- No intracerebral filling should be detected at the level of entry of the carotid or vertebral artery to the skull.
- The external carotid circulation should be patent.
- The filling of the superior longitudinal sinus may be delayed.

Electroencephalography

- A minimum of eight scalp electrodes should be used.
- Interelectrode impedance should be between 100 and 10,000.
- The integrity of the entire recording system should be tested.
- The distance between electrodes should be at least 10 cm.
- The sensitivity should be increased to at least $2\,\mu V$ for 30 minutes with inclusion of appropriate calibrations.
- The high—frequently filter setting should not be set below 30 Hz, and the low—frequently setting should not be above 1 Hz.
- Electroencephalography should demonstrate a lack of reactivity to intense somatosensory or audiovisual stimuli.

Transcranial Doppler ultrasonography

- There should be bilateral insonation. The probe should be placed at the temporal bone above the zygomatic arch or the verte-brobasilar arteries through the suboccipital transcranial window.
- The abnormalities should include a lack of diastolic or reverberating flow and documentation of small systolic peaks in early systole. A finding of transtemporal windows for insonation.

Cerebral scintigraphy (technetium Tc 99m hexametazime)

- The isotope should be injected within 30 minutes after its reconstitution.
- A static image of 500,000 counts should be obtained at several time points: immediately, between 30 and 60 minutes later, and at 2 hours.
- A correct intravenous injection may be confirmed with additional images of the liver demonstrating uptake (optional).

Brain death is a clinical diagnosis. A repeat clinical evaluation 6 hours later is advised (option), but a firm recommendation cannot be given and the interval is arbitrary. A confirmatory test is not mandatory in most situations. All clinical tests are needed to declare brain death and are likely equally essential. (One should not prioritize individual brain stem tests.) A confirmatory test is needed for patients in whom specific components of clinical testing cannot be reliably evaluated.

GUIDELINES FOR THE DIAGNOSIS OF BRAIN DEATH BY CANADIAN MEDICAL ASSOCIATION

Canadian Congress of Neurological Science. Guidelines for the diagnosis of Brain Death endorsed by Canadian Medical Association. CMAG Vol. 136. Jan 15, 1987.

Guidelines

The clinical diagnosis of brain death can be made when all the following criteria have been satisfied.

1. An etiology has been established that is capable of causing brain death and potentially reversible conditions have been excluded.
2. The patient is in deep coma and shows no response within the cranial nerve distribution to stimulation of any part of the body. No movements such as cerebral seizures, dyskinetic movements, decorticate or decerebrate posturing arising from the brain are present.
3. Brain stem reflexes are absent.
4. The patient is apneic when taken off the respirator for an appropriate time.
5. The conditions listed above persist when the patient is reassessed after a suitable interval.

Comments

Although the purpose of this document is to state general principles and recommended guidelines rather than to outline a set of rules, certain features of the guidelines merit more detailed explanation.

1. Cessation of brain function. The clinical absence of brain function is defined as profound coma, apnea and the absence of brain stem reflexes.

Coma: The patient should be observed for spontaneous behavior and response to noxious stimuli. In particular, there should be no motor response within the cranial nerve distribution to stimuli applied to any body regions. There should be no spontaneous or elicited movements (dyskinesias, decorticate, or decerebrate posturing or epileptic seizures) arising from the brain. However, various spinal reflexes may persist in brain death.

Brain stem reflexes: Pupillary light and corneal, vestibulocular and pharyngeal reflexes must be absent. The pupils should be midsize or larger and must be unreactive to light. Care should be taken that atropine or related drugs that could block the pupillary response to light have not been given to the patient. The vestibulo-ocular reflexes should be tested with caloric stimulation while the head is 30 degree above the horizontal. In adults a minimum of 120 ml of ice water should be used. Grimacing or any other motor response to pharyngeal or tracheal suctioning is incompatible with brain death.

Apnea was originally defined as lack of respiration when the patient was disconnected from the respirator for 3 minutes. This failed to consider whether an adequate $PaCO_2$ level was present to trigger respiration. The $PaCO_2$ threshold for respiratory stimulation in comatose patients in respirators have low $PaCO_2$ levels that rise slowly (e.g. 2 to 3 mmHg/min) when the respirator is stopped. In patients who fulfill the other clinical criteria of brain death, apneic oxygenation, described below, is a safe way of testing respiratory activity.

If blood gas determinations are available, the $PaCO_2$ should be 40+/−5 mmHg before testing for apnea begins. The patient should be preoxygeneted 9 L/mm (but not hyperventilated) with 100% oxygen for 10 minutes before testing. The respirator is then disconnected for 10 minutes, while to prevent hypoxemia, 100% oxygen is delivered at 6 L/mm, through an endotracheal cannula. This should produce a sufficient rise in $PaCO_2$ to serve as a respiratory stimulant.

If blood gas determination are not available, and adequate test of brain stem responsiveness to hypercarbia can be provided by ventilating the patient for 10 minutes, with a 95% oxygen 5% carbon dioxide mixture before the 10-minute apneic oxygenation. In patients with severe respiratory disease, it is advisable to obtain the opinion of a respiratory physician to determine the safety and validity of this test for apnea. Testing for apnea without passive oxygenation is not recommended. In addition to its potential deleterious effects on the brain, the resultant hypoxemia can occasionally cause complex movements of the limbs and trunk, presumably owing to spinal cord ischemia, that could be confused with reflex movements of cerebral origin.

2. Irreversibility: Cessation of brain function is determined to be irreversible when potentially reversible causes have been excluded and the changes are judged to be permanent. Drug intoxication (particularly of barbiturates, sedatives and hypnotics), treatable metabolic disorders, hypothermia (core temperature less than 32.2°C). Shock and peripheral nerve or muscle dysfunction due to disease or neuromuscular-blocking drugs must be excluded. Re-evaluation is essential to ensure that the non-functioning state of the brain is persistent and to reduce the possibility of observer error. Depending on the etiology, the interval between such examinations may be as short as 2 hours or as long as 24 hours. Observation for at least 24 hours is usually recommended to confirm brain death due to anoxia/ischemia (e.g. post-cardiac arrest). In situations where brain death is declared for purposes of organ transplantation, local regulations may stipulate specific intervals for reassessment.

Special Circumstances

1. Infants and children. Brain death has not been sufficiently well studied in neonates, infants and young children to determine whether clinical criteria listed above apply to these groups.
2. Inability to apply the clinical criteria. Some clinical situations such as uncertainty regarding etiology, inability to examine one or both eyes due to trauma, middle ear injuries, cranial neuropathies or severe pulmonary disease

may preclude the valid application of the listed clinical criteria. In these circumstances, the only reliable means of confirming brain death is the absence of cerebral perfusion determined by cerebral angiography or radionuclide scintigraphy.

Laboratory Test

Although brain death can be established reliably by clinical criteria alone, special tests can be used to support and in some instances supplement the clinical diagnosis. The electro-cephalogram assesses cerebral cortical function. Electro-cerebral inactivity is confirmation of brain death only if all the clinical criteria apply, and established techniques are followed to ensure proper sampling of cortical activity. Visual auditory and somatosensory evoked responses or other tests may eventually prove to be useful, but at present, there are no standard guidelines for their use in assessing patients with suspected brain death. The absence of intracranial perfusion, demonstrable by cerebral angiography or radionuclide scintigraphy, is reliable evidence of brain death. The mean arterial pressure should be greater than 80 mmHg when cerebral perfusion is assessed. If cerebral angiography or radionuclide scintigraphy is used to determine the absence of cerebral perfusion, the procedure should be performed by an appropriately qualified specialist.

The above set of guidelines was prepared by a sub-committee of the Canadian Congress of Neurological Sciences and has been approved by the membership of the Canadian Neurological Society, the Canadian Neurosurgical Society, the Canadian Association for Child Neurology and the Canadian Society of Clinical Neurophysiologist.

EUROPE

In Denmark and Great Britain the brain stem criteria is used. In the other countries brain death has to be demonstrated. Some countries have laws, other medical guidelines.

In England the first report was made in a conference of Medical Royal College and Faculties, which resulted in a report published in British Medical Journal in 1976.[49]

Holland has taken a leading position in the liberal legacy of transplantation. Both cadaveric transplantations as well as transplantations from brain dead persons are performed. Due to the excellent organ perfusion medias the organs to be transplanted can overcome longer and longer periods of cold ischemia. When a person is brought dead to the emergency care unit in a Dutch hospital, IV lines are administered to the patient and perfusion with organ preservation medias are given until the staff has contacted the family to orient about the death and request the permission for organ donation. This is also the case in patient where resuscitation is not successful.

In Holland organ removal is only allowed with the consent of the donor given in his lifetime or with the consent given from the next of kin. This is also the case in Great Germany, Denmark, Sweden and Turkey. In all the other European countries, that have a law concerning organ donations, and not just medical guidelines, there is the principle of presumed consent. In Belgium and France there are registers for objections such as national registers in Belgium and hospital registers in France. In Austria the removal of organs from a brain dead without any obligation to consult or inform the next of kin. This regulation is also applied to foreigners who die in Austria.

SCANDINAVIA

In Denmark brain death is defined as brain stem death with irreversible apneic-coma with absent brain stem reflexes. The clinical examination has to be conducted twice by two different doctors, who each have to do it twice with at least one hour interval between each examination. The doctors may do the examination together. One of the physicians has to be a specialist in neurology, neurophysiology or neurosurgery. If this is not possible whole brain death might be diagnosed by a 4-vessel angiogram repeated after 15 minutes. This must not show any intrathecal blood flow. These guidelines are only used in cases where permission has been given for a patient to donate organs. Otherwise, the mechanical ventilation is discontinued to stop a meaningless and useless treatment of a patient.

In Norway a 4-vessel angiogram is required but only if the patient is going to be an organ donor. The time of death is the time, where the 4-vessel examination is concluded. If the patient is not to become a donor the mechanical ventilation is stopped after one clinical brain stem death examination.

In Sweden no cerebral angiographies are required to verify brain death. If the patient is to be an organ donor, two clinical brain stem death examinations are carried out with an interval of 2 hours. Only one doctor is required, which means that one doctor can perform the examination twice. The time of death is the time, where the second brain stem death examination is accomplished.

THE UK CODE

Conditions for Considering Brain Death

All the following should coexist:

1. The patient is deeply comatose
   - Exclude the presence of cerebral depressant drugs, particularly if hypothermia is present or there is a history of drug injection.
   - Exclude hypothermia, body temperature should be at least 35 degree centigrade.
   - Exclude abnormalities of metabolism or endocrine system. In particular abnormalities of serum electrolytes, acid–base balance, blood sugar.
2. The patient is being maintained on a ventilator because spontaneous respiration had previously become inadequate or had ceased altogether. Exclude presence of muscle relaxant drugs or other respiratory depressants.
3. There should be no doubt that the patient's condition is due to irremediable structural brain damage. The diagnosis of a disorder which can lead to brain death should have been fully established.

Tests for confirming brain death are given as follows.

All Brain Stem Reflexes Should be Absent

1. The pupils are fixed in diameter and do not respond to sharp changes in the intensity of incident light.

2. There is no corneal reflex.
3. The vestibulo-ocular reflexes are absent. These are absent when no eye movement occurs during or after the slow injection of 20 ml of ice-cold water into each auditory meatus in turn. Clear access to the tympanic membrane must have been established by direct inspection. This test may be contraindicated by local trauma.
4. No motor responses within the cranial nerve distribution can be elicited by adequate stimulation of any somatic area.
5. There is no gag reflex response to bronchial stimulation by a suction catheter passed down the trachea.
6. No respiratory movements occur when the patient is disconnected from the mechanical ventilator long enough to ensure that pCO_2 rise above 6.7 kPa. Blood gases should be measured and recorded. Patients with preexisting chronic respiratory disease may be unresponsive to raised pCO_2 and exist on a hypoxic drive to respiration. These cases must be carefully evaluated with blood gas measurements.

Recommended Procedure

1. Pre-oxygenate with 100% oxygen for 5 minutes.
2. Take and record arterial blood gas sample.
3. Disconnect patient from the ventilator for up to 6 min to enable the $PaCO_2$ to rise at least 6.7 kPa (50 mmHg). Maintain oxygenation by in sufflation of oxygen at 8.1/min.
4. Take and record arterial blood gas sample. As an alternative the $PaCO_2$ can be raised to the required level by pre-ventilation with 5% carbon dioxide in oxygen before the ventilator is disconnected.

Other Considerations

Integrity of Spinal Reflexes

Spinal reflexes can persist after irretrievable destruction of brain stem function and may be present in brain dead patients.

Confirmatory Investigations

Electroencephalography, cerebral angiography or cerebral blood flow measurements are not necessary to diagnose brain death.

Body Temperature

Must be above 35°C before tests are carried out.

Specialist Opinion and Status of Doctors Concerned

The diagnosis of brain death should be made by two medical practitioners who have expertise in this field. Clinicians with wide experience of intensive therapy or acute medicine should not need specialist advice, but if there is any doubt it is necessary to consult a neurologist or neurosurgeon.

One of the two must be a consultant, the other a consultant or senior registrar who should assure themselves that the preconditions have been met before testing is carried out. The length of time required before preconditions can be satisfied varies according to circumstances, and although occasionally it might be less than 24 hours. It may extend to several days.

The two doctors may carry out the tests separately or together. If the tests confirm brain death they should nevertheless be repeated. There may be circumstances in which it is impossible or inappropriate to carry out one of the tests. The criteria published by the conference given recommended guidelines rather than rigid rules and it is for the doctors at the bedside to decide when the patient is dead.

Repetition of Testing

It is customary to repeat the tests to ensure that there has been no observer error. The interval between tests varies with the diagnosis and clinical course of the disease. It is common in practice to allow 24 hours to elapse, but this interval might be very much less and no particular time is suggested in the statement. It is for the two doctors to decide how long the interval between tests should be, but the time should be adequate for the reassurance of all those directly concerned. At the conclusion of each set of tests, each doctor must record their findings on the form that is available in all hospitals in the UK. This record must be attached to the patient's notes.

JAPAN

In Japan the brain death criteria is not yet taken into use. The only transplantations performed are those from live donors.

In 1985 the following statement was published.

Criteria for brain death by the Ministry of Welfare Brain Death research group:

1. Deep coma (3 by the Glasgow Coma Scale)
2. Lack of spontaneous respiration (Apnea test is indispensable)
3. Mydriasis of both pupils (24 mm).
4. Lack of brain stem reflexes (pupils to light, corneal reflexes, cough reflex). Lack of spontaneous movements, decorticate or decrebrate rigidity, convulsions must be excluded.
5. Flat EEG.
6. Re-testing after 6 hours interval.

Essentials

1. Organic brain damage.
2. Deep coma, apnea.
3. Verification of causative disease.
4. No evidence of recovery.

Exclusions

1. Children under the age of 6 years.
2. Diseases mimicking brain death (acute drug intoxicants, metabolic and endocrinological disorder, hypothermia).

The judgement must be performed by more than two doctors having experience with this test.

The criteria is only about brain death. No statement is made if the brain death is the death of the individual. Only live family transplantations are permitted.

These are only diagnosis about the functional status. The evidence about complete suspension of cerebral blood flow may be indispensable.

CHINA

In China there is extensive organ donor programs. China also has planned organ transplantations after executions of prisoners.

INDIA

The Transplantation of Human Organs Act 1994 in India (Act No. 42 of 1994)

(Received the assent of the President on 8-7-1994. Act published in Gaz. of India; 11-7-1994, Part II-S.1, Ext., P.I. (No. 58). (8th July, 1994).

Courtesy: Mr X Felix, Advocate, High Court.

An act to provide for the regulation of removal, storage and transplantation of human organs for therapeutic purposes and for the prevention of commercial dealings in human organs and for matters connected therewith or incidental thereto.

Whereas it is expedient to provide for the regulation of removal storage and transplantation of human organs for therapeutic purposes and for the prevention of commercial dealings in human organs:

And whereas Parliament has no power to make laws for the states with respect to any of the matters aforesaid except as provided in Articles 249 and 250 of the constitution.

And whereas in pursuance of CI. (1) of Article 252 of the constitution, resolutions have been passed by all the Houses of the Legislatures of the States of Goa, Himachal Pradesh and Maharashtra to the effect the matters aforesaid should be regulated in those States by Parliament by law:

Be it enacted by the Parliament in the forty-fifth year of the republic of India as follows.

Preliminary

I. Short title, application and commencement:

1. This act may be called the Transplantation of Human Organs Act, 1994.
2. It applies for the first instance, to the whole of the states of Goa, Himachal Pradesh (Maharashtra) and to all the

Union Territories and it shall apply to other states which adopts this act by resolution passed in the behalf under Clause (i) of Article 252 of the constitution.

3. It shall come into force in the states of Goa, Himachal Pradesh and Maharashtra and in all the union territories on such date as the Central Government may, by Notification, appoint and in any other state which adopts this act by resolution passed in that behalf under Clause (I) of Article 252 of the constitution. On the date of such adoption; and any reference in this act to the commencement of this act shall, in relation to any state or union territory means the date on which this act comes into force in such state or union territory.

II. Definitions: In this act, unless the context otherwise requires.

a. "advertisement includes any form of advertising whether to the public generally or to any section of the public or individually to selected persons."

b. "Appropriate Authority" means the appropriate authority appointed under Section 13.

c. "Authorization Committee" means the committee constituted under Clause (a) or Clause (b) of Subsection (4) of Section 9.

d. "Brain-stem death" means the stage at which all functions of the brain stem have permanently and irreversibly ceased and is so certified under Subsection (6) of Section 3.

e. "Deceased person" means a person in whom permanent disappearance of all evidence of life occurs, by reason of brain stem death or in a cardiopulmonary sense, at any time after live birth has taken place.

f. "Donor" means any person, not less than eighteen years of age, who voluntarily authorizes the removal of any of his human organs for therapeutic purposes under Subsection (I) or Subsection (2) of Section 3.

g. "Hospital" includes a nursing home, clinic, medical centre, medical or teaching institution for therapeutic purposes and other like institution.

h. "Human organ" means any part of human body consisting of a structured arrangement of tissues which if wholly removed, cannot be replicated by the body.

i. "Near relative" means spouse, son, daughter, father, mother, brother or sister.

j. "Notification" means any notification published in the Official Gazette.

k. "Payment" means payment in money or money's worth but does not include any payment for detraying or reimbursing.

   I. The cost of removing, transporting or preserving the human organ to be supplied; or

   II. Any expenses or loss of earnings incurred by a person so far as reasonably and directly attributable to his supplying any human organ from his body.

   III. "Prescribed" means prescribed by rules made under this Act.

l. "Recipient" means a person into whom any human organ is or is proposed to be transplanted;

m. "Registered medical practitioner" means a medical practitioner who possesses any recognized medical qualification as defined in Clause (h) of Section 2 of the Indian Medical Council Act. 1956, and who is enrolled on a State Medical Register as defined in Clause (k) of that section.

n. "Therapeutic purposes" means systematic treatment of any disease or the measure to improve health according to any particular method or modality; and

o. "Transplantation" means the grafting of any human organ from any living person or deceased person to some other living person for therapeutic purposes.

III. Authority for removal of human organs

1. Any donor may, in such manner and subject to such conditions as may be prescribed, authorize the removal, before the death of any human organ of his body for therapeutic purposes.

2. If any donor, in writing and in the presence of two or more witnesses (at least one of whom is a near relative of

such person), unequivocally authorized at any time before his death, the removal of any human organ of his body, after his death, for therapeutic purposes, the person lawfully in possession of the dead body of the donor shall, unless he has any reason to believe that the donor had subsequently revoked the authority aforesaid, grant to a registered medical practitioner all reasonable facilities for the removal, for therapeutic purposes, of that human organ from the dead body of the donor.

3. Where no such authority as is referred to in Subsection (2), was made by any person before his death but no objection was also expressed by such person to any of his human organs being used after his death for therapeutic purposes, the person lawfully, in possession of the dead body of such person may be, unless he has reason to believe that any near relative of the deceased person has objection to any of the deceased person's human organs being used for therapeutic purposes, authorize the removal of any human organ for the deceased person for its use for therapeutic purposes.

4. The authority given under Subsection (1) or Subsection (2) or, as the case may be, Subsection (3) shall be sufficient warrant for the removal, for therapeutic purposes of the human organ; but no such removal shall be made by any person other than the medical practitioner.

5. Where any human organ is to be removed from the body of a deceased person, the registered medical practitioner shall satisfy himself, before such removal, by a personal examination of the body from which any human organ is to be removed, that life is extinct in such body or, where it appears to be a case of brain stem death, that such death has been certified under Subsection (6).

6. Where any human organ is to be removed from the body of a person in the event of his brain stem death, no such removal shall be undertaken unless such death is certified, in such form and in such manner and on satisfaction of such manner and on satisfaction of such conditions and requirements as may be prescribed, by a Board of medical experts consisting of the following, namely:

I. The registered medical practitioner in charge of the hospital in which brain stem death has occurred;

II. An independent registered medical practitioner, being a specialist, to be nominated by the registered medical practitioner specified in clause (i) from the panel of names approved by the appropriate authority.

III. A neurologist or a neurosurgeon to be nominated by the registered medical practitioner specified in clause (i), from the panel of names approved by the appropriate authority; and

IV. The registered medical practitioner treating the person whose brain stem death has occurred.

7. Notwithstanding anything contained in Subsection (3), where brain stem death of any person, less than eighteen years of age, occurs and is certified under Subsection (6), and of the parents of the deceased person may give authority, in such form and in such manners as may be prescribed, for the removal of any human organ from the body of the deceased person.

IV. Removal of human organs not be authorized in certain cases

1. No facilities shall be granted under Subsection (2) of Section 3 and no authority shall be given under Subsection (3) of that section for the removal of any human organ from the body of a deceased person. If the person required to grant such facilities, or empowered to give such authority, has reason to believe that an inquest may be required to be held in relation to such body in pursuance of the provisions of any law for the time being in force.

2. No authority for the removal of any human organ from the body of a deceased person shall be given by a person to whom such body has been entrusted safely for the purpose interment, cremation or other disposal.

V. Authority for removal of human organs in case of unclaimed bodies in hospital or prison:

1. In the case of dead body lying in a hospital or prison and not claimed by any of the near relatives of the deceased

person within forty-eight hours from the time of the death of the concerned person, the authority for the removal of any human organ from the dead body which so remains unclaimed may be given, in the prescribed form, by the person in charge, for the time being, of the management or control of the hospital or prison or by an employee of such hospital or prison authorized in this behalf by the person in charge of the management or control hereof.

2. No authority shall be given under Subsection (i) if the person empowered to give such authority has reason to believe that any near relative of the deceased person is likely to claim the dead body even though such near relative has not come forward to claim the body of the deceased person within the time specified in Subsection (1).

VI. Authority for removal of human organs from bodies sent for post-mortem examination for medico-legal or pathological purpose. Where the body of a person has been sent for post-mortem examination:

a. For medical-legal purposes by reason of the death of such person having been caused by accident or any other unnatural case;

or

b. For pathological purposes.

The person competent under this act to give authority for the removal of any human organ from such dead body, if he has reason to believe that such human organ will not be required for the purpose for which such body has been sent for post-mortem examination, authorize the removal, for therapeutic purposes of that human organ of the deceased person provided that he is satisfied that the deceased person had not expressed, before his death, any objection to any of the human beings used, for therapeutic purposes after his death, or, where he had granted an authority for the use of any of his human organs for therapeutic purposes, after his death, such authority had not been revoked by him before his death.

VII. Preservation of human organs: Saving after the removal of any human organ from the body of any person, the registered medical practitioner shall take such steps for the preservation of the human organ so removed as may be prescribed.

VIII. (1) Nothing in the foregoing provisions of the act shall be constructed as rendering unlawful any dealing with the body or with any part of the body of a deceased person if such dealing would have been lawful if this act not been passes.

(2) Neither the grant of any facility of authority for the removal of any human organ from the body of a deceased person in accordance with the provisions of this act nor the removal of any human organ from the body of any deceased person in pursuance under Section 297 of the Indian Penal Code.

IX. Restrictions on removal and transplantation of human organs

1. Save as otherwise provided in Subsection (3), no human organ removed from the donor before his death shall be transplanted into a recipient unless the donor is a near relative of the recipient.

2. Where any donor authorizes the removal of any of his human organs after his death under Subsection (2) of Section 3 or any person competent or empowered to give authority for the removal of any human organ from the body of any deceased person authorizes such removal, the human organs may be removed and transplanted into the body on any recipient who may be in need of such human organ.

3. If any donor authorizes the removal of any of his human organ before his death under Subsection (1) of Section 3 for transplantation into the body of such recipient, not being a near relative, as is specified by the donor by reason of affection or attachment towards the recipient or for any other special reasons, such human organ shall not be removed and transplanted without the prior approval of the Authorization Committee.

4. (a) The Central Government shall constitute, by Notification, one or more Authorization Committees consisting of such members as may be nominated by the

Central Government on such terms and conditions as may be specified in the notification for each of the Union territories for the purposes of this section.

(b) The State Government shall constitute, by Notification, one or more Authorization Committees consisting of such members as may be nominated by the State Government on such terms and conditions as may be specified in the notification for the purposes of this section.

5. On an application jointly made, in such form and in such manner as may be prescribed by the donor and the recipient, the Authorization Committee shall, after holding an inquiry and after satisfying itself that the applicants have complied with all the requirements of this act and the rules made hereunder, grant to the applicants approval for the removal and transplantation of the human organ.

6. If, after the inquiry and after giving an opportunity to the applicants of being heard, the Authorization Committee is satisfied that the applicants have not complied with the requirements of this act and the rules made thereunder, it shall for reasons to be recorded in writing, reject the application for approval.

X. Regulation of hospitals conducting the removal, storage or transplantation of human organs:

1. On and from the commencement of this act:
   a. No hospital, unless registered under this act, shall conduct, or associate with, or help in, the removal, storage or transplantation of any human organ;
   b. No medical practitioner or any other person shall conduct, or cause to be conducted, or aid in conducting by himself or through any other person, any activity relating to the removal, storage or transplantation of any human organ at a place other than a place registered under this act, and
   c. No place including a hospital registered under Subsection (1) of Section 15 shall be used or cause to be used by any person for the removal, storage or transplantation of any human organ except for therapeutic purposes.

2. Notwithstanding anything contained in Subsection (1), the eyes or the ears may be removed at any place from the dead body of any donor, for therapeutic purposes, by a registered medical practitioner.

Explanation: For the purposes of this subsection, "ears" includes ear drums and ear bones.

XI. Prohibition of removal or transplantation of human organs for any purpose other than therapeutic purposes: No donor and no person empowered to given authority for the removal of any human organ shall authorise the removal of any human organ for any purpose other than therapeutic purposes.

XII. Explaining effects, etc. to donor and recipient: No registered medical practitioner shall undertake the removal or transplantation of any human organ unless he has explained, in such manner as may be prescribed, possible effects, complications and hazards connected with the removal and transplantation to the donor and the recipient respectively.

XIII. Appropriate Authority:
1. The Central Government shall appoint, by notification, one or more officers as appropriate authorities for each of the union territories for purposes of this act.
2. The State Government shall appoint, by notification, one or more officers as appropriate authorities for this purpose of this act.
3. The appropriate authority shall perform the following functions, namely:
   i. To grant registration under Subsection (1) of Section 15 or renew registration under Subsection (3) of that section;
   ii. To suspend or cancel registration under Subsection (2) of Section 16;
   iii. To enforce such standards, as may be prescribed, for hospitals engaged in the removal, storage or transplantation of any human organ;
   iv. To investigate any complaint to breach of any of the provisions of this act or any of the rules made thereunder and take appropriate action;

v. To inspect hospitals periodically for examination of the quality of transplantation and the follow-up medical care to persons who have undergone transplantation and persons from whom organs are removed; and

vi. To undertake such other measures as may be prescribed.

XIV. Registration of hospitals engaged in removal, storage or transplantation of human organs:

1. No hospital shall commence any activity relating to the removal, storage or transplantation of any human organ for therapeutic purposes after commencement of this act unless such hospital is duly registered under this act;

   Provided that every hospital engaged, either partly or exclusively, in any activity relating to the removal, storage or transplantation of any human organ for therapeutic purposes immediately before the commencement of this act, shall apply for registration within sixty days from the date of such commencement;

   Provided further that every hospital engaged in any activity relating to the removal, storage or transplantation of any human shall cease to engage in any such activity on the expiry of three months from the date of commencement of this act unless such hospitals have applied for registration and is so registered or till such application is disposed of, whichever is earlier.

2. Every application for registration under Subsection (1) shall be made to the appropriate authority in such form and in such manner and shall be accompanied by such fees as may be prescribed.

3. No hospital shall be registered under this act unless the appropriate authority is satisfied that such hospital is in a position to provide such specialized services and facilities, possess such skilled manpower and equipments and maintain such standards as may be prescribed.

XV. Certificate of registration:

1. The appropriate authority shall, after holding an inquiry and after satisfying itself that the applicant has complied

with all the requirements of this act and the rules made thereunder, grant to the hospital a certificate of registration in such form, for such period and subject to such conditions as may be prescribed.

2. If, after the inquiry and after giving an opportunity to the applicant of being heard, the appropriate authority is satisfied that the applicant has not complied with the requirements of this act and the rules made thereunder, it shall, for reasons to be recorded in writing, reject the application for registration.

3. Every certificate of registration shall be, renewed in such manner and no payment of such fees as may be prescribed.

XVI. Suspension or cancellation of registration:

1. The appropriate authority may, suo motu or on complaint, issue a notice to any hospital to show cause why its registration under this act should not be suspended or cancelled for the reasons mentioned in the notice.

2. If, after giving a reasonable opportunity of being heard to the hospital, the appropriate authority is satisfied that there has been a breach of any of the provisions of this act or the rules made thereunder it may, without prejudice to any criminal action that it may take against such hospital, suspend its registration for such period as it may think fit or cancel it registration.

   Provided that where the Appropriate Authority is of the opinion that it is necessary or expedient so to do in the public interest, it may for reasons to be recorded in writing, suspend the registration of any hospital without issuing any notice.

XVII. Appeals: Any person aggrieved by an order of the Authorisation Committee rejecting an application for approval under Subsection (6), of Section 9, or any hospital aggrieved by an order of the Appropriate Authority rejecting an application for registration under Subsection (2) of Section 15 or an order of suspension or cancellation of registration under Subsection (2) of Section 16, may within thirty days from the date of the receipt of the order, prefer an appeal, in such manner as may be prescribed, against such order to.

1. The Central Government where the appeal is against the order of the Authorisation Committee constituted under Clause (a) of Subsection (4) of Section 9 or against the order of the appropriate authority appointed under Subsection (1) of Section 3; or

2. The State Government, where the appeal is against the order of the Authorisation Committee constituted under Clause (b) of Subsection (4) of Section 9 or against the order of the appropriate authority appointed under Subsection (2) of Section 13.

XVIII. Punishment for removal of human organs without authority:

1. Any person who renders his services to or at any hospital and who, for the purposes of transplantation, conducts, associate with, or helps in any manner in the removal of human organ without authority, shall be punishable with imprisonment for a term which may extend for 5 years or a fine which may extend up to Rs. 10,000.

2. Where any person convicted under Subsection (1) is a registered medical practioner, his name shall be reported by appropriate authority to the respective State Medical Council for taking necessary action including the removal of his name from the register of the council for a period of 2 years for the first offence and permanently for the subsequent offence.

XIX. Punishment for commercial dealings in human organs whoever:

a. Makes or receives any payment for the supply of, or for an offer to supply any human organ;

b. Seeks to find a person willing to supply for payment any human organ;

c. Offers to supply any human organ for payment;

d. Initiates or negotiates any arrangement involving the making of any payment for the supply of, or for an offer to supply any human organ;

e. Takes part in the management or control of a body of persons, whether a society, firm or company, whose activities consist of or include the initiation or negotiation of any arrangement referred to in Clause (d); or

f. Publishes or distributes or causes to be published or distributed an advertisement,

    i. Inviting persons to supply for payment of any human organ;

    ii. Offering to supply any human organ for payment; or

    iii. Indicating that the advertiser is willing to initiate or negotiate any arrangement referred to in Clause (d);

        Shall be punished with imprisonment for a term which shall not be less than 2 years but which may extend to 7 years and shall be liable to fine which shall not be less than Rs. 10,000 but may extend to Rs. 20,000.

Provided that the court may, for any adequate and special reason to be mentioned in the judgement, impose a sentence of imprisonment for a term of less than 5 years and a fine of less than Rs. 5,000.

XX. Punishment for contravension of any other provision of this act—whoever contravenes any provision of this act on any rule made, or any condition of the registration granted, thereunder for which no punishment is separately provided in this act, shall be punishable with imprisonment for a term which may extend to 3 years or with a fine which may extend to Rs. 5,000.

XXI. Offences by Companies:

1. Where any offence, punishable under this act has been committed by a company, every person who, at the time the offence was committed was in charge of, and was responsible to the company for the conduct of the business of the company, as well as the company shall be deemed to be guilty of the offence and shall be liable to be proceeded against and punished accordingly.

    Provided that nothing contain in this subsection shall render any such person liable to any punishment, if he proves that the offence was committed without his knowledge or that he had exercised all due diligence to prevent the commission of such offence.

2. Notwithstanding anything contained in Subsection (1), where any offence punishable under this act has been committed by a company and it proved that the offence has been committed with the consent or connivance of, or is attributable to any neglect on the part of, any director, manager, secretary or other officer shall also be deemed to be guilty of that offence and shall be liable to be proceeded against and punished accordingly.

Explanation for the purpose of this section.

a. "company' means any body corporate and includes a firm or other association of individuals, and

b. "director", in relation to firm, means a partner in the firm.

XXII. Cognizance of offences:

1. No court shall take cognizance of an offence under this act except on a complaint made by:
   a. The appropriate authority concerned, or any officer authorized in this behalf by the central government or the state government or, as the case may be, the appropriate authority; or
   b. A person who has given notice of not less than sixty days, in such manner as may be prescribed, to the appropriate authority concerned, of the alleged offence and of his intension to make a complaint to the court.

2. No court other than that of a metropolitan magistrate or a judicial magistrate of the first class shall try any offense punishable under this act.

3. Where a complaint has been made under Clause (b) of Subsection (1), the court may, on demand by such person, direct the appropriate authorities to make available copies of the relevant in its possession to such person.

Miscellaneous

XXIII. Protection of action taken in good faith

1. No suit, prosecution or other legal proceedings shall lie against any person for anything which is in good faith

done or intended to be done in pursuance for this provisions of this act.

2. No suit or other legal proceeding shall be against the central government or the state government for any damage caused or likely to be caused for anything which is in good faith done or intended to be done in pursuance for the provisions of this act.

XXIV. Power to make rules:

1. The central government may, by notification, make rules for carrying out the purposes of this act.

2. In particular and without prejudice to the generally of the foregoing power, such rules may provide for all or any of the following matters, namely:

   a. The manner in which and the conditions subject to which any donor may authorize removal before his death, of any human organ of his body under Subsection (1) of Section 3;

   b. The form and the manner in which a brain stem death is to be certified and requirements which are to be satisfied for that purpose under Subsection (6) of Section 3;

   c. The form and the manner in which any of the parents may give authority, in the case of brain stem of a minor for the removal of any human organ under Subsection (7) of Section 3;

   d. The form in which authority for the removal of any human organ from an unclaimed dead body may be given by the person in charge of the management or control of the hospital or prison, under Subsection (1) of Section 5;

   e. The steps to be taken for the preservation of the human organ removed from the body of any person under Section 7;

   f. The form and the manner in which the application may be jointly made by the donor and the recipient under Subsection (5) of Section 9;

g. The manner in which all possible effects, complications and hazards connected with the removal transplantation is to be explained by the registered medical practioner to the donor and the recipient under Section 12;

h. The standards as are to be enforced by the appropriate authority for the hospitals engaged in the removal, storage or transplantation of any human organ under Clause (iii) of Subsection (3) of Section 13;

i. Other measures as the appropriate authority shall undertake in performing its functions under Clause (vi) of Subsection (3) of Section 13;

j. The form and the manner in which an application for registration shall be accompanied, under Subsection (2) of Section 14.

k. The specialized services and the facilities to be provided skilled manpower and equipment to be possessed and the standards to be maintained by a hospital for registration, under Subsection (3) of Section 14;

l. The form in which, the period for which and the conditions subject to which certificate of registration is to be granted to a hospital, under Subsection (1) of Section 15;

m. The manner in which and the fee on payment of which certificate of registration is to be renewed under Subsection (3) of Section 15;

n. The manner in which an appeal may be preferred under Section 17.

o. The manner in which a person is required to give notice to the appropriate authority of the alleged offence and of his intention to make a complaint to the court under Clause (b) of Subsection (i) of Section 22, and

p. Any other matter which is required to be or may be prescribed.

3. Every rule made under this act shall laid, as soon as may be after it is laid before each house of Parliament while it is in session for a total period of 30 days which may be

comprised in 1 session or in 2 or more successive sessions and if, before the expiry of the section immediately following the section or the successive sessions aforesaid, both houses agree that the rule should not be made, the rule shall thereafter have effect in such modified form or be of no effect as the case may be; so however, when any such modification or annulment shall be without prejudice to the validity of anything previously done under that rule.

XXV. Repeat and savings:

1. The Ear Drums and Ear Bones (Authority for Use for Therapeutic Purposes) Act, 1982 and the Eyes (Authority for Use for Therapeutic Purposes) Act, 1982 are hereby repealed.
2. The repeat shall, however, not affect the previous operation of the acts so repeal or anything duly done or suffered thereunder.

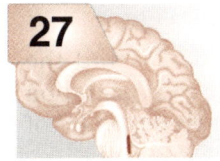

27

Outline the International Brain Stem Death Protocol

The phenomenon brain death or brain stem death is universal. Brain stem death is not one thing in one part of the world and another thing in another part of the world. Brain stem death is irreversible apneic-coma with brain stem areflexia. The clinical implication of this condition will unequivocally lead to death whether or not mechanical ventilation is carried on for a period of time. In patients where the brain stem death criteria is fulfilled, mechanical ventilation can thus be stopped and the individual as a whole will die due to cardiac arrest. These patients may be potential organ donors, and for this reason the mechanical ventilation can be carried out until the organs that are to be donated are removed. But this is only a question of hours—not days. For this reason an international unanimous clinical brain stem death code is proposed to be used internationally.

Brain Stem Death Protocol

Patient data: Name and hospital number (sticker) Date:

A. Cause of coma: _____

B. Has 6 hours passed since the time of irreversible brain stem ischemia:

C. Suspicion of any reversible conditions that could have caused coma?

     Neuromuscular agents given: _____

     Sedative agents (last dose given): _____

     Hypothermia: _____ Date _____ Time

     Metabolic or endocrine disturbances: _____

D. Clinical brain stem examination:

(In case of absence of all reflexes, examination to be repeated after one hour).

     1. Do the pupils react to light?   _____ _____

     2. Are there corneal reflexes?   _____ _____

     3. Is the oculo-cephalic reflex present?   _____ _____

     4. Is the vestibule-ocular reflex present?   _____ _____

     5. Is there any reaction to pain in the face? _____ _____

     6. Is the gag reflex present?   _____ _____

     7. Is the cough reflex present?   _____ _____

     8. Is the cilio-spinal reflex present?   _____ _____

     9. Is there any reaction to pain stimulus? _____ _____

     10. Is there spontaneous respiration?   _____ _____

E. Result of apnea test (PaCO$_2$)   _____ _____

F. Time of death (2nd PaCO$_2$)   _____ _____

G. Examination by _____

Name, signature and position of examining physician.

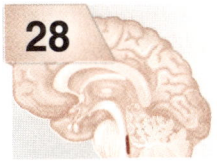

28   What is Lazarus Syndrome?

When the mechanical ventilation is stopped in a patient who is declared brain stem dead, and the heart slowly ceases to beat, it is sometimes seen that the patients start to move. In the old days these moving phenomenon in dying patients were well-known, because the family used to be around the dying patient, and everybody knew that old unconscious patients suddenly could have some bright movements at last, uttering a few words and rising a bit up from the bed. These phenomena have also been described in the medical literature concerning brain death. Jordan Alter in 1985 writes: "There is even a Lazarus-sign where patients 5–10 minutes after the ventilator has been stopped show sudden movements of the arms and shoulders". Ropper in 1984[172] describes one patient who 5 minutes after respiratory support was stopped and cardiac function ceased, crossed both arms over his chest and began to sit up.

The physician call this spinal reflexes due to mechanical and hypoxic stimuli, which probably tricker the upper cervical cord motor neurons to produce these signs. Even though physicians explain these movements by medical terms such as persistent spinal cord reflexes, a biblical name has been chosen for the syndrome. The syndrome of Lazarus is taken from the Bible hinting to the resurrection of Lazarus from the dead.

29   What are the Steps to be Followed When a Diagnosis for Brain Death is Being Considered?

1. Testing

   a. The first test to be done by the consultant of ICU unit.

b. The second series of test to be done by two consultants of the department, one of whom should be on the officially nominated panel.

c. The second series to be done 6 hours after the first.

2. Ensure that the following results are available (or at least have been sent) at the conclusion of the first series of tests:

a. Blood for Hepatitis B surface antigen

b. Blood for HIV

c. Blood for HCV

d. Blood for blood group analysis

e. Blood for liver function tests

f. Blood for WBC TC/DC

g. Blood for PT, PTT and platelets

3. Inform transplant coordinator about possible candidate after first positive test. (*Note:* The protocol is to be aborted if the transplant team examines the candidate, enquires about the candidate or talks to the candidate's relatives before this.)

4. The coordinator will

a. Interact with family and keep the ICU informed at all times.

b. Inform all other personnel of the transplant team (it is not the responsibility of the ICU to contact anyone other than the coordinator).

c. Obtain all drugs and fluids necessary for the patient once the first test is positive.

d. Complete all legal formalities except for filling Form 8.

5. The time of death in all cases will be recorded as the time of the second positive test.

FORM-8

[See rule a(3)(a)and (b) of the THO Rules 1995]

We, the following members of the Board of medical experts after careful personal examination, hereby certify that

Shri/smt./km ....

Aged about ....

S/o, d/o, w/o, Shri ....

Resident of ....

.... is dead on account of permanent and irreversible cessation of all functions of the brain stem. The tests carried out by us and the findings therein are recorded in the brain stem death certificate annexed hereto.

Dated ....   Signature ....

1. R.M.P., Incharge of the hospital in which brain stem death has occurred
2. R.M.P., nominated from the panel of names approved by the appropriate authority
3. Neurologist/Neuro-surgeon nominated from the panel of names approved by the appropriate authority
4. R.M.P., treating the aforesaid deceased person

BRAIN STEM DEATH CERTIFICATE

Patient Details:

1. Name of the patient   Shri/smt/km. ....

   ....

   SO/DO/WO   Shri . ...

   ....

   Sex .... Age ....

2. Home address ....
   ....
   ....

3. Hospital number ....

4. Name and address of next of ....
   kin or person responsible for the ....
   patient (if none exists, this must ....
   be specified) ....
   ....
   ....

5. Has the patient or next of kin ....
   agreed to any transplant? ....
   ....

6. Is this a police case? Yes.................... No ....

Pre-conditions

1. Diagnosis: Did the patient suffer from any illness or accident that led to irreversible brain damage? Specify details.
   ....
   ....
   ....

   Date and time of accident/onset of illness ....
   Date and onset of non-responsive coma ....

2. Findings of board of medical experts:

i. The following reversible causes of coma have been excluded: Intoxication (alcohol)
   Depressant drugs
   Relaxants (neuromuscular blocking agents)

	First Medical Examination		Second Medical Examination	
	1st	2nd	1st	2nd

Primary hypothermia

Hypovolemic shock

Metabolic or

    endocrine disorders

Tests for absence of

    brain stem functions

ii. Coma

iii. Cessation of spontaneous breathing

iv. Papillary size

v. Pupillary light reflexes

iv. Doll's head eye movements

vii. Corneal reflexes (both sizes)

viii. Motor response in any cranial nerve distribution, any responses to stimulation of face, limb or trunk

ix. Gag reflex

x. Cough (tracheal)

xi. Eye movements on coloric testing bilaterally

xii. Apnea tests as specified

xiii. Were any respiratory movements seen?

....

Date and time of first testing :

....

This is to certify that the patient has been carefully examined twice after an interval of about six hours and on the basis of findings recorded above. Shri/Smt/Km. .... Is declared brain stem dead

1. Medical Administrator incharge   2. Authorised specialist
   of the hospital
3. Neurologist/Neuro-surgeon   4. Medical Officer treating the patient

NB. I. The minimum time interval between the first testing and second testing will be six hours.

    II. No. 2 and No. 3 will be co-opted by the administrator incharge of the hospital from the panel of experts approved by the appropriate authority.

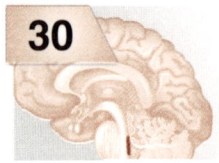

30

What are the Pitfalls in the Diagnosis of Brain Death?

Findings	Possible causes
1. Pupils fixed	Anticholinergic drugs Neuromuscular blockers Preexisting disease
2. No oculovestibular reflexes	Ototoxic agents Vestibular suppressants Preexisting disease
3. No respiration	Posthyperventilation apnea Neuromuscular blockers
4. No motor activity	Neuromuscular blockers "Locked-in" state Sedative drugs
5. Isoelectric EEG	Sedative drugs Anoxia Hypothermia Encephalitis Trauma

Potential pitfalls accompany the diagnosis of brain death, particularly when coma occurs in hospitalized patients or those who have been chronically ill. Almost none of these will lead to serious error in diagnosis if the examining physician is aware of them and attends to them when examining individual patients who are considered brain dead. Some of these pitfalls are outlined above.

In comatose patients, pupillary fixation does not always mean absence of brain stem function. In rare instances, the pupils may have been fixed by preexisting ocular or neurologic disease. More commonly, particularly in a patient who has suffered cardiac arrest, atropine has been injected during the resuscitation process and widely dilated, fixed pupils may result without indicating the absence of brain stem function. Neuromuscular blocking agents also can produce pupillary fixation, although in these instances the pupils are usually midposition or small rather than widely dilated.

Similarly, the absence of oculovestibular responses does not necessarily indicate absence of brain stem vestibular function. Like pupillary responses, oculovestibular reflexes may be present if the end organ is either poisoined or damaged. Some otherwise neurologically normal patients suffer labyrinthine dysfunction from peripheral disease that predates the onset of coma. Other patients with chronic illnesses have suffered ototoxicity from a variety of drugs, including antibiotics such as gentamicin. In these patients, oculovestibular responses may be absent even though brain stem processes are still functioning. Finally, a variety of drugs, including sedatives, anticholinergics, anticonvulsants, and tricyclic antidepressants, may suppress vestibular and/or oculomotor function to the point where oculovestibular reflexes disappear.

Pitfalls also exist in the diagnosis of apnea in comatose patients maintained on respirators.

The absence of motor activity also does not guarantee loss of brain stem function. Neuromuscular blockers are often used early in the course of artificial respiration when the patient is resisting the respirator; if suspected brain death subsequently occurs, there may still be enough circulating neuromuscular blocking agent to produce absence of motor function when the examination is carried out. A recent report has described the stimulation of brain death by excessive sensitivity to succinylcholine. In this case the presence of activity in the EEG established cerebral viability.

Therapeutic overdoses of sedative drugs to treat anoxia or seizures likewise may abolish reflexes and motor responses to noxious stimuli.

There are pitfalls in using the EEG as an ancillary technique in the diagnosis of cerebral death. Isoelectric EEGs with subsequent recovery have been reported with sedative drug overdoses, after anoxia, during hypothermia, following cerebral trauma, and after encephalitis.

The three cardinal findings in brain death are coma or unresponsiveness, absence of brain stem reflexes, and apnea.

PITFALLS CAN OCCUR AT EACH LEVEL

1. Motor Responses of the Limbs

Pitfalls: Motor responses ("Lazarus sign") may occur spontaneously during apnea testing, often during hypoxic or hypotensive episodes, and are of spinal origin. Neuromuscular blocking agents can produce prolonged weakness. If neuromuscular blocking agents have recently been administered, examination with a bedside peripheral nerve stimulus should result in four thumb twitches.

2. Pupils

Pitfalls: Many drugs can influence pupil size, but light response remains intact. In conventional doses, atropine given intravenously has no marked influence on pupillary response. A report of fixed, dilated pupils after extremely high doses of dopamine has not been confirmed.

Because nicotine receptors are absent in the iris, neuromuscular blocking drugs do not noticeably influence pupil size. Topical ocular instillation of drugs and trauma to the cornea or bulbus oculi may cause abnormalities in pupil size and can produce nonreactive pupils. Preexisting anatomic abnormalities of the iris or effects of previous surgery should be excluded.

3. Ocular Movements

Pitfalls: Drugs that can diminish or completely abolish the caloric response are sedatives, aminoglycosides, tricyclic antidepressants, anticholinergics, antiepileptic drugs, and chemotherapeutic agents. After closed head injury or facial trauma, lid edema and chemosis of the conjunctiva may restrict movement of the globes. Clotted blood or cerumen may diminish the caloric response, and repeat testing is required after direct inspection of the tympanum. Basal fracture of the petrous bone abolishes the caloric response only unilaterally and may be identified by an ecchymotic mastoid process.

4. Facial Sensation and Facial Motor Response

Pitfall. Severe facial trauma may limit interpretation of all brain stem reflexes.

5. Pharyngeal and Tracheal Reflexes

Pitfall. In orally intubated patients, the gag response may be difficult to interpret.

Clinical observations compatible with the diagnosis of brain death.

Respiratory acidosis hypoxia, or brisk neck flexion may generate spinal cord responses.

Spontaneous movements of the limbs from spinal mechanisms can occasionally occur and more frequent in young adults. These spinal reflexes include rapid flexion in arms, raising of all limbs off the bed, grasping movements, spontaneous jerking of one leg, walking-like movements and movements of the arms up to the point of reaching the endotracheal tube.

Respiratory-like movements may also occur and are typical agonal breathing patterns. They are characterized by shoulder elevation and adduction, back arching, and inter-costal expansion without any significant tidal volume.

Other responses are profuse sweating, blushing, tachycardia, and sudden increases in blood pressure. These hemodynamic responses can sometimes be elicited by neck flexion, and they can be eliminated by ganglion blockers (e.g. Trimethaphan). Normal blood pressure and absence of diabetes insipidus without pharmacologic support are compatible with brain death. Muscle stretch reflexes, superficial abdominal reflexes, and Babinski reflexes are of spinal origin and do not invalidate a diagnosis of brain death. Patients may have initial plantar flexion of the great toe followed by sequential brief planter flexion of the second, third, fourth and fifth toes after snapping of one of the toes (undulating "toe flexion sign").

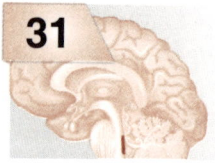

31

Is it Possible to Predict Which Comatose Patients will Progress to Brain Death?

It is not possible to determine with confidence which comatose patients will progress to brain death, even though several studies have identified the clinical parameters associated with a poor neurologic outcome. The best predictor or neurologic outcome is the level of brain stem function observed within the first 24 hours after presentation. The lack of pupillary response to light on initial exam is a very poor prognostic sign. By 72 hours after cerebral insult, the motor response to pain increases in predictive value, with absent or posturing response to pain excluding the possibility of independent neurologic recovery.

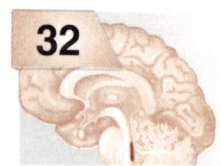

32

Briefly Summarize Brain Death Criteria

NEUROLOGICAL EXAMINATION

Fixed dilated or intermediate size pupils with absent light reflex.

- Absent corneal reflex
- Absent oculocephalic reflex
- Absent oculovestibular reflex
- Absent gag reflex
- Non-spontaneous during apnea test
- No reaction to deep central pain
- Absence of conditions that could stimulate brain death
- Hypothermia, hypoxia, drugs, hypotension, metabolic
- Aetiology of brain death must be clearly established

Observation Period

Neurological examination must not be done within thirty minutes following CPR.

If structural brain damage has been demonstrated, another neurological examination is performed 6 hours, after the first one compatible with brain stem death otherwise the second neurological examination is performed 24 hours after the first one.

Paraclinical Confirmatory Test

No paraclinical confirmatory test is required if the previous points are fulfilled.

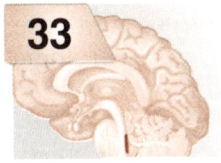

33

Who Should Declare Brain Death?

Not only neurologists and neurosurgeons, but also intensivists anesthesiologist, and other specialists staffing intensive care units and emergency departments are gaining expertise and experience in this area, and their ability in regard to this diagnosis should be recognized. General medical curricula and testing of physician qualifications should encompass brain death. Anyone with competence should be able to make this diagnosis. A computerized algorithm has been developed in Germany to guide the declaration and clarity problems.

Some criteria (and state laws) suggest that two physicians must agree on the diagnosis of brain death, particularly when organ retrieval is being considered. If an electrocephalogram is done, the electroencephalographer may be the second physician. However, if the diagnosis is straightforward and clear, and if the physician involved is experienced and well trained. It would seem reasonable for a single physician to certify brain death.

Once a patient is declared brain dead, support could legally be terminated. Some believe that the physician has the authority and the responsibility to stop the respirator and other life-sustaining treatment when a patient is dead and that the option to continue care should not be given to the family. Others believe that physicians should ask families for permission to stop care and turn off the respirator. In any case, when managing distraught or otherwise difficult families, it is prudent to listen for and consider objections. The question may arise in these circumstances as to whether one must continue to employ all possible life-sustaining treatment for the patient.

Many families may benefit from a short period of time to adjust to the sudden tragedy and hopelessness of the situation. They may need this opportunity to develop trust in their physician and the diagnosis. If the family objects to discontinuation of the respirator, particularly because of family stress or religious reasons, it may be wisest to delay until the family dynamics are clarified and family members feelings can be addressed. However, the physician should not mislead the family by implying any insecurity regarding the diagnosis and the fact that the patient is dead. Problems arise when a family becomes distrustful or irrational. A consultant may be called. Chaplains and ministers as well as ethics committees may be helpful in aiding such families. When brain death has been caused by criminal assault, thoughtful legal advice becomes essential.

That followed by Govt of Tamil Nadu is as follows: G.O. (Ms) No. 75, G.O. (Ms) No. 6, Health and Family Welfare Department Dated 8.1.2008

Form 8 of the THO Act and Rules as found in the Annexure I to this order are prescribed as the brain death certification format to be utilised for any given situation requiring certification that a person is dead on account of permanent and irreversible cessation of all functions of the brain stem. The tests prescribed therein and the findings required shall remain the same.

According to Form 8 of the said Act and Rules, when such certification is required, there shall be two medical examinations conducted by a team of doctors after a minimum interval of six hours and the findings made based on the tests prescribed therein.

One aspect of the above form requires further clarification and this is provided in Annexure II of this order.

According to Form 8 of the above Act and Rules, four doctors are authorised to certify brain death and this provision is clarified further.

(A) Doctor No. 1 is the 'RMP in charge of the hospital in which brain stem death has occurred'. Accordingly, the Registered Medical Practitioner in charge of the hospital in which brain stem death has occurred shall refer to either the Head of the Institution, RMO, ARMO, duty RMO or the RMP in charge of the Hospital. (No clearance is required from the appropriate authority in this category.)

(B) Doctor No. 2 is the 'RMP (physicians, surgeons or intensivists) nominated from the panel of names approved by the appropriate authority'. Accordingly, a panel of names shall be sent by the Dean/Medical Superintendent/Medical Director to the approprate authority, namely the Director of Medical and Rural Health Services and on approval shall then be utilised as the panel from which a RMP shall be nominated for each brain death certification. Each hospital may determine its own procedure for this duty.

(C) Doctor No. 3 is 'Neurologist/Neuro-surgeon nominated from the panel of names approved by the appropriate authority'. Again, a panel of names shall be sent by the Dean/Medical Superintendent/Medical Director to the appropriate authority, namely the Director of Medical and Rural Health Services and on approval shall then be utilised as the panel from which one specialist as in the category therein shall be nominated for each brain death certification. Each hospital may determine its own procedure for this duty.

(D) Doctor No. 4 is the RMP treating the aforesaid person. This does not require any clarification and shall be the RMP/Doctor on duty treating the patient. (No clearance is required from the appropriate authority in this category.)

Note: (i) In the event of lack of authorised personnel in Category 3 above in the hospital concerned, a request may be made to any other member of the panel from another hospital.

(ii) The 1st and 2nd medical examination as defined in Form 8 of the THO rules shall be conducted by category 2 and 3 doctors from the panel approved by the appropriate authority.

Although it has been made mandatory for the three medical college hospitals in Chennai to follow this procedure, the same procedure shall be applicable to all hospitals inclusive of private hospitals which wish to certify brain death as and when required. Accordingly, the categories that require for the panel to be approved shall be done so on submission to the appropriate authority (Director of Medical and Rural Health Services.)

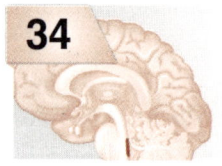

34

How to Maintain Brain Dead Patients?

Appropriate support before and after brain death can improve the number and quality of donor organs. Donor management is a continuation of previous critical care management but with a shift in goals. It should be delivered in intensive care staff by experienced staff.

GOALS OF ORGAN DONOR MANAGEMENT

- Maintain body temperature
- Adequate oxygenation
- . Adequate circulating volume
- Cardiovascular stability
- Adequate urine output

I. To follow "Rule of 100"
Systolic arterial pressure >100 mmHg
Urine output >100 ml/hour
PaO_2 >100 mmHg
Hg Conc >100 g/lit
Blood sugar 100% normal

II. Main aim is directed at optimizing transplantable organ function. High quality critical care including chest physiotherapy, aseptic precautions and antibiotics may be required.

III. Primary goals are maintenance of adequate tissue perfusion and preservation of organ viability.

DURATION OF DONOR MANAGEMENT

If high quality donor management was available, delaying transplantation to improve donor condition is acceptable. The approach is "relax and repair" rather than "rush and retrieve". When the donor is stable retrieval should be started since there is a risk of deterioration if retrieval is delayed.

The actual timing of retrieval depends on which organs are likely to be retrieved and whether other organs will be transplanted even if function improved.

> **Key point**
>
> Prolonged cold ischemic time certainly has an adverse effect on the function of all transplanted organs particularly hearts. Planning must limit cold ischemic time and allow optimal timing for recipient operations.

Common Medical Problems in Brain Dead Patient

Hypotension
Coagulopathy
Diabetes insipidus
Cardiac ischemia (i.e. arrhythmias)
Renal failure
Acute lung injury
Acute respiratory distress syndrome

SUMMARY OF THE PRINCIPLES OF DONOR MANAGEMENT

General Care

i. Management in intensive care unit (facilities required nursing and medical care and support of relatives).
ii. Continued invasive monitoring.
iii. Adherence to infection control procedures.

   iv. Mouth and eye care

   v. Hygiene needs as required

   vi. Regular patient repositioning

   vii. Nursing with the head of the bed elevated to reduce the risk of aspiration.

Respiratory

1. 'Lung protective' ventilation. Tidal volume 6–8 ml/kg with optimal PEEP to allow minimum FiO_2.
2. Recruitment manoeuvres to be maintained.
3. Maintain tracheal cuff pressure at 25 cm H_2O.
4. Avoid overload with fluids.

Cardiovascular

1. Accurate fluid balance
2. Correct hypovolemia—colloids preferred over isotonic saline.
3. Since vascular tone is impaired cardiac output monitoring may be needed to titrate fluids or pressor drugs to intended goals as guided by retrieval team.
4. Dose of vasopressin 0–2.4 units/hr (DA VP, 1-deamino-8-D-arginine. Vasopressin)
5. High doses of catecholamines (e.g. Norepinephrine >0.05 μg/kg/min.) should be avoided if possible.
6. Consider tri-iodothyronine bolus and infusion. Dose: 4 μg bolus then infusion at 3 $μg/h^{-1}$ or levothyroxine

Fluids

a. Administer maintenance fluid (can use enteral route). But avoid positive balance and hyponatremia.

b. Monitor urine output—0.5–2.5 ml/kg/hr

   If urine output is >4 ml/kg/hr consider diagnosis of diabetes insipidus and treat with vasopressin infusion or DDVAP.

Nutrition

1. Insulin infusion 1 unit/hr minimum
2. Maintain feeding or glucose source. Blood glucose target 4–8 mmol/lit (80–160 mg%)
3. Electrolyte abnormalities to be corrected to normal values

Blood and Coagulation

1. Correct coagulation if evidence of active bleeding
2. Consider need for coagulation support during retrieval
3. Consider need for transfusion
4. Maintain thromboprophylaxis as there is high incidence of pulmonary emboli found at retrieval.

Steroids

Methyl prednisolone 15 mg/kg bolus immediately after brain death confirmed.

Investigations

1. Full blood count
2. Urea, creatinine, electrolytes
3. Liver enzymes, INR, PT, PPT
4. Blood glucose
5. ABG
6. Culture–blood, urine, sputum
7. ECG
8. Echocardiogram
9. Coronary angiogram may be indicated
10. Bronchoscopy and lavage followed by lung recruitment manoeuvres
11. Chest X-ray after lung recruitment procedure

To increase the number of organs that meet the criteria for transplantation, the medical care of the potential organ donor must be protective and aggressive.

MONITORING OF ORGAN DONOR

Optimal hemodynamic management requires invasive monitoring.

> **Key points**
>
> 1. Because of the order in which great vessels are ligated during the operation, any newly placed arterial cannula should be inserted into the left radial or brachial artery.
> 2. A new central venous or pulmonary artery catheter (PAC) should be inserted into the right internal jugular or subclavian veins.
> 3. Intravenous fluid administration must be carefully monitored as organs, particularly the lungs are susceptible to volume overload and capillary leakage.

Echocardiography is useful to exclude major structural abnormalities of the heart and to measure left ventricular ejection fraction if it is less than 45%, then insertion of PA catheter may be helpful.

Transthoracic echocardiography (TTE) may be technically difficult and better images may be obtained with trans-oesophageal echocardiography (TOE). Transient regional wall motion abnormalities, systolic inward motion and thickening may improve with hemodynamic optimization.

Assessment of right ventricular size and function is important and frequently challenging.

Temperature Support

Hypothermia should be anticipated and heat loss prevented by using

- Warmed intravenous fluids
- Warming blankets
- Heated and humidified inspired gases
- Increased ambient temperature

STANDARD DONOR CARE

1. Blood pressure, heart rate, temperature, urine output, central venous pressure (CVP) [If central venous

catheter present], pulmonary artery occlusion pressure (PAOP) [if pulmonary artery (PA) catheter is present] q1 hour

2. Reorder mechanical ventilator parameters as previously set

3. Maintain head of bed at 30–40 degrees elevation

4. Continue routine pulmonary suctioning and side-to-side body positioning

5. Warming blanket to maintain body temperature above 36.5°C

6. Maintain sequential compression devices (SCDs)

7. [If present] continue chest tube suction or water seal as previously ordered

8. [If present] nasogastric (orogastric) tube to low intermittent suction

9. Intravenous fluid—D5 0.45% saline plus 20 meq KCL per liter at 75 cc/hour.

10. Call ICU incharge if: MAP<70 mm Hg; systolic pressure >170 mmHg; Heart rate<60>130 bpm; Temp <36.5°C>37.8°C; urine output<75>250 cc/hr; CVP or PAOP<8>18 mmHg

11. Medications: Pantoprazole 40 mgm IV q24 hours, artificial tears q1 hour to prevent corneal drying albuteral and atrovent unit dose per aerosol q4 hours continue antibiotics previously ordered at same dose and frequency. Continue vasoactive drug infusions (dopamine, norepinephrine, etc) at previously ordered concentrations and infusions rates. [Review all medications previously ordered.]

   Most (anticonvulsants, pain medications, laxatives, gastrointestinal motility agents, eye drops, antihypertensives, anti-nausea agents, subcutaneous heparin, osmotic agents (mannitol), and diuretics) are unnecessary during donor care and will be discontinued automatically when declared brain dead. [Review any other medications in question with MD.]

12. Send electrolytes, magnesium, ionized calcium, CBC, platelets, glucose, blood urea nitrogen, creatinine,

phosphorus, arterial blood gas, prothrombin time (PT), partial thromboplastin time.

13. Finger stick glucose q2 hours—call, if glucose <90>180 mgm/dl
14. electrocardiogram STATs
15. Chest X-ray indication: Initial donor evaluation
16. Add other orders for specific organ evaluation as indicated.

The above order set provides a "safety net" of call orders so that the ICU incharge is alerted to significant changes in donor status. It also prescribes the foundation for ongoing monitoring of physiological and laboratory variables.

Donor care is subsequently directed and "fine-tuned" through the guidelines that follow. These include treatment plans for hypertension, hypotension, glucose management, temperature, anemia, coagulopathy and thrombocytopenia, mechanical ventilation, fluid and electrolyte treatment, polyuria, and acid–base changes. Each may be referenced as that circumstance/problem arises. Although the guidelines are not intended to compartmentalize the complex process of overall donor care, they may be helpful in providing useful resources in methods of treatment, precautions, and points at which MD consultation is appropriate.

Guideline—Hypertension

Introduction: It is unusual for hypertension to occur after brain death, although it is common during the evolution of brain death. Because donor organs are likely at more risk from hypotension than hypertension, a conservative treatment plan is recommended. The goal for mean arterial blood pressure (MAP) is <90 mmHg when the donor is hypertensive, but always above 65–70 mmHg. The MAP is measured via an intra-arterial catheter, non-invasive blood pressure device or calculated by: Diastolic pressure + 1/3 (systolic–diastolic pressure) +5. Therapy should be started if the MAP is sustained above 95 mmHg for 30 minutes after certification of brain death. Placement of the arterial catheter in an upper extremity is preferred.

Treatment

A. Reduce or discontinue inotropic or vasopressor medications or infusions

B. If the difference between the MAP recorded via an arterial catheter and non-invasive machine is >20 mmHg—discuss which blood pressure to follow with the physician—consultant (MD). Differences in measurements take from an automatic oscillometric non-invasive device and an arterial catheter may be due to several technical factors.

C. Give labetalol 20 mgm IV bolus every 20 minutes until MAP goal (65–70 mmHg) is reached. If the MAP goal is not achieved after 2 doses begin infusion.

D. NTG infusion—start infusion at 5 mgm/hr and titrate up to 12 mgm/hr to achieve the MAP goal.

E. If the MAP goal is not achieved after titration of NTG to 15 mgm/hr, consult MD.

Guideline—Hypotension

Introduction

Hypotension commonly follows brain death and may be caused by on-going or pre-existing conditions leading to hemorrhagic, cardiogenic, distributive, or obstructive types of "shock". In the absence of these pre-existing conditions causing shock, hypotension commonly occurs after brain death due to loss of vasomotor centers in the brain causing vasodilation, decreased contractility of the heart, or hypovolemia due to ongoing fluid loss due to diabetes insipidus. Hypotension will be defined as a mean arterial blood pressure (MAP) of <60 mmHg as measured from an indwelling arterial catheter, non-invasive blood pressure machine, or calculated by: diastolic pressure+ 1/3 [systolic—diastolic pressure]. Placement of an arterial line for monitoring is desirable, and insertion in an upper extremity is preferred. The treatment goal for MAP is 65–75 mmHg.

Assessment

A. Review medical record for evidence of recent blood loss. Confirm that the most recent hematocrit (HCT) is >28%

and reaffirm with an immediate repeat HCT—Refer to guidelines—anemia and coagulopathy and treat as indicated if HCT<28% or a coagulation disorder is present.

B. Review medical record for evidence of concomitant myocardial ischemia/infarction during this admission. Repeat ECG and maintain at bedside. Consult MD for ECG interpretation.

C. Review medical record for evidence of excessive fluid losses above intake (output>intake by >1500 cc in last 24 hours) during current hospitalization. If polyuria is present, refer to guideline—polyuria.

D. Review current patient status for a central venous line and evaluate central venous pressure (CVP) or pulmonary artery (PA) catheter and evaluate pulmonary artery occlusion pressure (PAOP). The goal is to maintain both at 12–15 mmHg. If PA catheter present, obtain information regarding cardiac output, cardiac index, systemic vascular resistance index, and left ventricular stroke work index.

E. Review the medical record for evidence of ongoing severe infection, drug or other allergic reactions (e.g. due to transfusion), pericardial effusion, or pneumothorax. Obtain a chest radiograph and consult MD for its interpretation.

Treatment Algorithm

A. Assure any sign of continuing hemorrhage (external, GI, urinary, abdominal, etc.) has been evaluated and interventions initiated.

B. Discontinue medications that may contribute to hypotension (e.g. antihypertensive, beta-blockers).

C. The general principle of treatment is to first assure that adequate intravascular volume (preload) is present as evidenced by a CVP and/or PAOP greater than 12 mmHg.

D. Begin treatment with a crystalloid solution such as 0.9% saline (normal saline) or Ringer's lactate. Colloid solutions may be added and may be preferable for repeated fluid challenges (5% albumin 250 or 500 ml). Thereafter either intropic or vasopressor medications will be infused and titrated to the MAP goal or other hemodynamic parameters. If a PA catheter is available or at any time is inserted, a cardiac/hemodynamic profile should be obtained. If the donor demonstrates a low systemic vascular resistance index (SVRI) (<1400 dyne.sec.m^2/cm^5) a vasopressor (e.g. norepinephrine, phenylephrine) is the vasoactive drug of choice and subsequently titrated to maintain the MAP>60 mmHg. If the left ventricular stroke work index (LVSWI) is low (<35 gm.m/m^2), a positive inotropic agent (e.g. dopamine, dobutamine) should be used. The algorithm below assumes that if the MAP, CVP, heart rate and PAOP goals are reached, vital signs will continue to be monitored. Vasoactive medications should be weaned and removed as soon as possible, while maintaining the MAP goal. Subsequent deviations from goal values may require return to the guidelines.

Guideline—Glucose Management

Introduction

Both hypoglycemia and hyperglycemia may harm donor organs. Measure serum glucose every 4 hours and obtain finger stick glucose (FSG) per glucometer every 2 hours unless as described below.

Hypoglycemia

(Treat <75 mg/dl)

- A. Give 1 pre-mixed syringe of 50% dextrose (D50).
- B. Repeat glucose or obtain finger-stick glucose in 30 minutes and repeat 50% dextrose if glucose <75 mg/dl.
- C. If laboratory or finger stick glucose remains <75 mg/dl after 2 doses of D50, consult MD.

Hyperglycemia

(Treat serum glucose >150 mg/dl)

- A. Assure glucose removed from all IV fluids/infusions unless required by pharmacy.

B. The algorithms below show a subcutaneous insulin unless sliding scale and a supplemental IV insulin regimen.

   Note: Give subcutaneous insulin no more often than every four hours. When supplemental IV insulin is also needed, give the IV insulin bolus prescribed by the IV sliding scale every hour after the hourly FSG. Stop IV insulin when the blood sugar drops below 250 mg/dl.

C. In summary, hyperglycemia is treated by first removing sources of exogenous glucose, followed by subcutaneous insulin per the above sliding scale every four hours. Supplemental IV insulin is given each hour thereafter only if the blood glucose remains above 225 mg/dl.

D. Glucose subcutaneous insulin sliding scale.

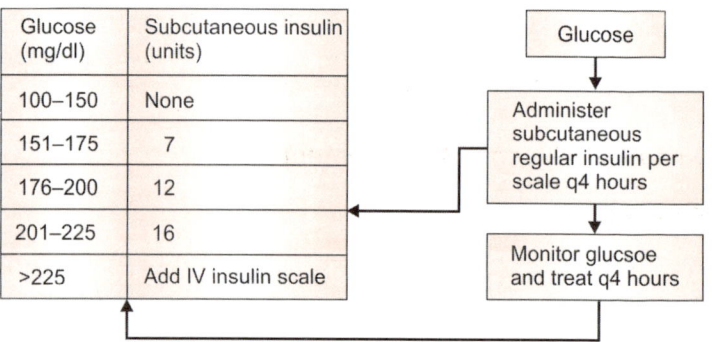

Glucose (mg/dl)	Subcutaneous insulin (units)
100–150	None
151–175	7
176–200	12
201–225	16
>225	Add IV insulin scale

E. Supplemental intravenous insulin sliding scale. Give the q4 hour subcutaneous insulin as prescribed above plus the hourly IV bolus prescribed below when the blood glucose of finger-stick glucose is >225 mg/dl.

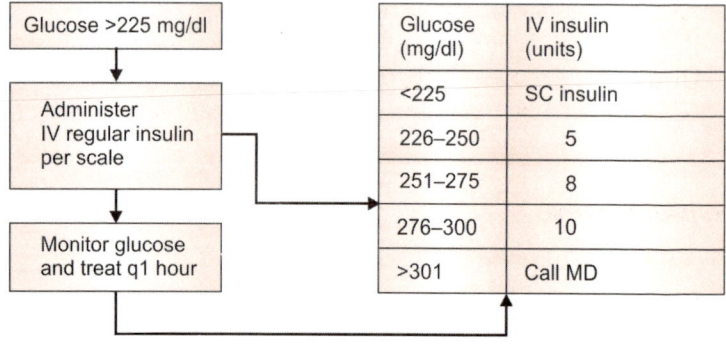

Glucose (mg/dl)	IV insulin (units)
<225	SC insulin
226–250	5
251–275	8
276–300	10
>301	Call MD

F. If glucose remains >250 mg/dl for hours after the initial subcutaneous insulin and subsequent IV insulin therapy, consult MD to discuss an insulin infusion.

Guideline—Temperature

Introduction

Brain death usually causes loss of thermal regulation in the donor, commonly resulting in hypothermia. The temperature goal is 36–37.5°C (97–99.5°F).

Hypothermia

(Treat <36°C (97°F))

A. The preferred method of body temperature measurement is from a core site, such as a pulmonary artery catheter or bladder (specialized catheter). Axillary temperatures should not be used, and oral temperatures are less accurate in hypothermia. Rectal temperatures can be used if hypothermia is not severe (>35°C).

B. Use active surface warming with a heated—liquid or hot air warming blanket plus insulating thermal blankets.

C. Warm the inspired gas from the ventilator to 38.5°C (101.3°F).

D. Minimize the amount of body surface and time of exposure to environmental temperatures.

E. If temperature remains <36°C after 3 hours of attempted re-warming, consult MD.

Hyperthermia

Unusual after brain death—treat >37.8°C (100.1°F).

A. Remove unnecessary blankets.

B. Do NOT cool inspired gas.

C. Acetaminophen 650 mgm per suppository or per gastric tube q3 hours.

D. Use automated fluid filled cooling blanket.

E. If temperature remains >101°F after 3 hours of cooling, consult MD.

Guideline—Anemia

Introduction

Although the differential diagnosis for anemia may be extensive, during donor care the most likely causes are continuing blood loss or excessive blood draws for laboratory testing. Hemolysis may rarely occur. The goal is to maintain the hematocrit (HCT) above 30%.

Assessment

A. Review medical record for evidence of bleeding sites, prior blood transfusions and their frequencies, or other information about blood loss or hemolysis.

B. Observe for signs of ongoing bleeding from:
  1. External wounds, IV sites, etc.
  2. GI tract via gastric tube or bowel movements; observe for abdominal distension and/or firmness and changes during repeat abdominal assessment.
  3. Urinary tract by observation or laboratory assessment for blood in count and treat as indicated.

C. Refer to Guideline—Coagulopathy. Obtain PT, PTT, fibrinogen and platelet count and treat as indicated.

D. If HCT 28–30% and no signs of bleeding are present begin q4 hr HCT measurements.

E. If HCT 28–30% and no gastric tube is in place, insert orogastric tube and lavage stomach to assess for upper GI blood.

Treatment

A. If prior transfusions have been required, submit blood bank order to maintain 2–4 units of packed red blood cells (PRBC) available. Otherwise, write order to type and cross-match and maintain 2 units PRBC available.

B. If HCT <30% transfuse 2 units PRBC rapidly.

C. Reassess HCT 1 hour after last unit PRBC infused and repeat transfusion if HCT <30%.

D. Reassess HCT 1 hour after 4th unit PRBC and reconsider above assessment items. If HCT <30% after 4 units PRBC, consult MD.

Guideline—Coagulopathy and Thrombocytopenia

Introduction

Blood loss from any cause may endanger continued perfusion to donor organs. Disseminated intravascular coagulation or a "dilutional" coagulopathy may occur after severe trauma and resuscitation. The treatment goal is to correct clinically important coagulopathy and thrombocytopenia. Because ongoing hemorrhage may worsen coagulation abnormalities and/or thrombocytopenia, refer to Guideline—Anemia, and correct disorders noted.

It is recognized that commonly performed laboratory tests of coagulation, i.e. partial thromboplastin time (PTT), prothrombin time (PT), fibrinogen, and the platelet count may be abnormal but treatment may not be required. Treatment is reserved for donors who appear to have continuing significant blood loss evidenced by physical assessment, hemodynamic instability and changes in coagulation parameters.

Assessment

A. The donor's medical record should be reviewed for any possible injury that may account for bleeding. If found— discuss with MD.

B. Review medical record to assure that no drugs that might interfere with coagulation or platelet function have recently been given, e.g. warfarin (Coumadin®), aspirin, heparin, clopidogrel (Plavix®), dypyridamole, etc. Notify MD if recent administration is documented.

C. Laboratory assessment—PT, PTT, fibrinogen, platelet count—repeat coagulation tests should be done 30 minutes after any administration of blood products.

Normal values: PT <14.5 seconds, platelet count >150,000/cc^3, PTT <35.6 seconds, fibrinogen: 150–350 mg/dl.

Measure ionized calcium—refer to Guideline—Fluid/ Electrolytes and treat hypoionized calcemia at <2.3/mEq/L (<1.2 mmol/L).

Treatment

Treatment of continued signs of significant blood loss and associated abnormal coagulation results or platelet count:

A. Consult MD for external bleeding or further assessment of possible GI or urinary injury. Treat anemia as per Guideline—Anemia.

B. Platelets—platelet dysfunction due to prior aspirin intake can be overcame by infusing a platelet 5-pack dose even though the platelet count is normal. Discuss with MD. Otherwise, treat for platelet count $<65,000/cc^3$.

   1. Transfuse 1 platelet pack (usually 5 or 6 individual units of platelets) intravenously as rapid infusion.

   2. Recheck platelet count one hour after first platelet pack and transfuse second platelet pack if platelet count remains $<65,000/cc^3$. Obtain follow-up platelet count exactly one hour after second platelet infusion completed.

   3. If platelet count remains $<65,000/cc^3$ after second platelet infusion, consult MD.

C. Coagulopathy **(Increased PT, PTT)**—treat PT>15 seconds, PTT >38 seconds

   1. If donor had been receiving intravenous heparin and PTT is >75 seconds, discuss administration of protamine with MD.

   2. Rapidly infuse 4 units fresh frozen plasma (FFP).

   3. Repeat PT, PTT measurements 30 minutes after initial FFP—repeat FFP if PT, PTT remain above treatment ranges.

   4. Repeat PT, PTT measurements 30 minutes after second FFP infusion—if PTT and PT remain elevated above treatment ranges, consult MD.

D. Coagulopathy **(Decreased fibrinogen)**—treat fibrinogen <100 mg/dl

   1. Infuse 6 units of cryoprecipitate, rapidly

   2. Repeat fibrinogen 1 hour after initial cryoprecipitate infusion—repeat infusion of cryoprecipitate if fibrinogen remains <100 mg/dl.

3. Repeat fibrinogen 1 hour after second infusion of cryoprecipitate. If concentration remains <100 mg/dl, consult MD.

Guideline—Mechanical Ventilation

Introduction

Under most circumstances volume limited controlled mechanical ventilation will be used during donor care. Pressure limited controlled mechanical ventilation is indicated when peak and plateau airway pressures are elevated, indicating high airway resistance or poor lung compliance (see below). The goals during mechanical ventilation are:

A. Peak airway pressure (Peak AWP) <40 cm H_2O
B. Plateau airway pressure (Plateau AWP) <35 cm H_2O
C. FIO_2—lowest possible to maintain SpO_2 >92% and PaO_2 >80 mmHg
D. PEEP—minimum 5 cm H_2O, adjust to maintain PaO_2 > 80 mmHg
E. Auto PEEP—<5 cm H_2O
F. Arterial blood gas (ABG) values: pH 7.35–7.45; $PaCO_2$ 36–44 mmHg to maintain pH within goal range; PaO_2 >80 mmHg; HCO_3 not independently adjusted.

Assessment

A. Evaluate the medical record for cardiopulmonary diseases prior to or during this admission. Assess related issues such as chronic oxygen use at home, ongoing pneumonia, chest radiograph results, culture results, antibiotics ordered, respiratory treatments given, etc.
B. Assure recent ABG results available or obtain sample for testing. Compare results to the above treatments goals.
C. Perform a physical examination with attention to abnormalities such as wheezing, Rhonchi, sputum appearance/ thickness/tenacity, etc.
D. Repeat ABGs at least every 4 hours or more frequently to assess changes in respiratory status or after adjustments in ventilator settings.

E. Consult with a respiratory care practitioner to identify if above mechanical ventilation goals are being met, i.e. auto PEEP, airway pressures, etc.

General Ventilator Settings

A. Volume—limited controlled ventilation

1. Tidal volume (VT)—10 ml/kg ideal body weight (kg). If high peak airway pressures are present, reduce VT to 6–8 ml/kg ideal body weight (kg).

   Ideal body weight:
   a. Male—50 kg + 2.3 kg per inch >60 inches
   b. Female—45 kg +2.3 kg per inch >60 inches

2. Rate (f)—adjusted to maintain minute ventilation (VT × f) (VE) of approximately 8–10 L/min or to maintain $PaCO_2$ >16 mmHg <60 mmHg, so as to maintain arterial pH at 7.35–7.45. Downward adjustment in rate may be needed to minimize auto PEEP.

3. Flow rate—usually about 60 L/min; adjust to minimize peak AWP; beware of auto PEEP as flow rate is slowed; higher flow rate may be needed to minimize auto PEEP.

4. PEEP—minimum 5 cm H_2O—adjusted to assist in maintaining PaO_2 >70 mmHg.

5. FIO_2—adjust to maintain PaO_2 >80 mmHg.

6. Use decelerating (ramp) pattern for flow delivery, when available.

B. Pressure—limited controlled ventilation

1. Inspiratory pressure setting—to limit peak airway pressure at 35–40 cm H_2O, consult with respiratory care practitioner for final pressure limit setting due to various ventilator types.

2. Rate—same as A(2) above

3. PEEP—same as A(4) above. However, recall PEEP adjustments may change delivered VT and VE during pressure—limited ventilation, i.e, increased PEEP will generally decrease VT and VE causing $PaCO_2$ to rise (reverse with decreased PEEP).

4. FIO_2—same as A(5) above.

General Respiratory Treatments

A. Assure adequate suctioning of excessive sputum.

B. Assure bronchodilators are ordered as indicated by wheezing or a peak airway pressure—plateau airway pressure gradient of >10 cm H_2O.

C. Other forms of chest physiotherapy or related devices are optional but should be considered.

Ventilator Adjustments—Volume-limited Controlled Ventilation

Note: Repeat ABG 30 minutes after any change of ventilator settings to assess effects.

Note: Combinations of adjustments listed below may be necessary as guided by arterial blood gas results and airway pressure.

A. Acidemic pH—arterial pH <7.35
   1. Increase VT to maximum 12 ml/kg ideal wt as long as plateau AWP remains <35 cm H_2O, or
   2. Increase rate to maximum 22 breaths/min as long as auto PEEP remains <5 cm H_2O
   3. If pH remains <7.32 after above changes, refer to treatment Guideline—Acid–Base treatment

B. Alkalemic pH—arterial pH >7.45
   1. Decrease ventilator rate sequentially to minimum of 6 breaths/min to achieve pH.
   2. Decrease VT to minimum of 6 ml/kg ideal body weight.
   3. If pH remains >7.45, consult MD.

C. High plateau AWP >35 cm H_2O
   1. Reduce flow rate to minimum 50 L/min—as long as auto PEEP remains <5 cm H_2O
   2. Reduce VT to minimum of 6 ml/kg ideal body wt—assess effect on arterial pH.
   3. Reduce PEEP to minimum 5 cm H_2O—assess effect on PaO_2.
   4. If plateau AWP remains >35 cm H_2O, consult MD.

D. Auto PEEP >5 cm H_2O
   1. Increase flow rate to maximum of 90 L/min—as long as plateau AWP remains <35 cm H_2O.
   2. Decrease VT to minimum 6 ml/kg ideal body wt—assess effect on arterial pH.
   3. Decrease ventilator rate sequentially to minimum of 8 breaths/min to minimize auto PEEP—assess effect on arterial pH.
   4. If auto PEEP remains >5 cm H_2O, consult MD.
E. Low PaO_2 <70 mmHg
   1. Increase FIO_2 to maximum 1.0 (100%).
   2. Increase PEEP to maximum 15 cm H_2O—as long as plateau AWP remains <35 cm H_2O.
   3. Add inspiratory pause (hold) to maximum 1.0 seconds as long as auto PEEP remains <5 cm H_2O.
   4. If PaO_2 remains <70 mmHg, consult MD.

Ventilator Adjustments—Pressure-limited Controlled Mechanical Ventilation

A. Acidemic pH—arterial pH <7.35
   1. Increase ventilator rate to maximum 22 breaths/min as long as auto PEEP <5 cm H_2O.
      Note: Auto PEEP will decrease VT delivered and may worsen acidemia.
   2. Increase inspiratory pressure setting to maximum peak AWP of 45 cm H_2O.
   3. If arterial pH remains <7.32, consult MD.
B. Alkalemic pH—arterial pH >7.45
   1. Decrease ventilator rate sequentially to minimum of 6 breaths/min to achieve pH goals.
   2. Decrease inspiratory pressure setting but maintain VT above 6 ml/kg ideal body wt.
   3. If arterial pH remains >7.45, consult MD
C. Auto PEEP >5 cm H_2O
   1. Decrease ventilator rate sequentially to minimum 8 breaths/min—assess effect on arterial pH.
   2. If >5 cm H_2O auto PEEP persists, consult MD.

D. Low PaO_2 <70 mmHg
1. Increase FIO_2 to maximum 1.0 (100%)
2. Increase ventilator PEEP to maximum of 15 cm H_2O as long as pH remains >7.35. (Increased PEEP will decrease tidal volume delivered in pressure-limited ventilation.)
3. If PaO_2 remains <70 mmHg, consult MD.

Guideline—Fluid Electrolyte Treatment

Introduction

The treatment goal is to maintain electrolytes within the normal limits established by the clinical laboratory in each hospital. To achieve that goal, laboratory testing phosphorous (P), and ionized Ca (Ca^{++}), should be completed every 4 hours. More frequent testing may be needed to monitor/treat critical levels. Any testing should be delayed for 30 minutes after the last dose of the electrolyte being treated. All electrolyte replacement should be by the intravenous route.

General Table of Normal Values

Na 136–142 mEq/L (mmol/L)   Mg 1.5–2.3 mg/L
(0.65–1.05 mmol/L)

K 3.5–5.0 mEq/L (mmol/L)   Phos 2.3–4.7 mg/dl
(0.74–1.52 mmol/L)

Cl 96–106 mEq/L (mmol/L)
Ionized Ca 2.3–2.54 mEq/L
HCO_3 21–28 mEq/L (mmol/L)   (1.15–1.27 mmol/L)

Electrolyte Therapy

A. **Sodium (Na)**
1. Hypernatremia—treat Na>150 mEq/L
a. With polyuria (>250 cc of urine above intake per hour)—see Guideline—Polyuria
b. Without polyuria—give 1 liter 0.2% saline as rapid infusion and replace urine output cc/cc/hr with 0.2% saline if pharmaceutically possible and that any

maintenance IV is D5% 0.2% saline. Avoid use of diuretics.

2. Hyponatremia—treat for serum Na <133 mEq/L

   a. Mix all medications in 0.9% saline (normal saline) if pharmaceutically possible. Change maintenance IV to D5 0.9% saline

   b. If hyperglycemia is present, the serum Na may be low because of the high blood glucose. If blood sugar >300, a "corrected" serum Na may be calculated by adding to the measured Na 1.6 mEq for each 100 gm/dl of blood glucose above 100. See Guideline—Hyperglycemia and treat.

   c. If Na <128 mEq/L give 3% NaCl per infusion (central line preferred) at 40 cc/hr × 3 hours.

   d. If Na remains <133 mEq/hr after 3% NaCl infusion, consult MD.

B. Potassium (K)

1. Hyperkalemia—treat serum K—5.8 mEq/L

   a. **Note:** Do not treat K if laboratory reports specimen "hemolyzed"—send a new specimen for testing.

   b. Assure all K removed from current infusions

   c. Repeat serum Kq1 hour

   d. Give IV:

      1. 50 cc of 50% dextrose (D50) (one pre-filled syringe)

      2. 15 units regular humulin insulin

      3. 1 amp $NaHCO_3$ (44 or 50 meq via pre-filled syringe)

   e. If K >5.8 mEq/L after above intervention, consult MD.

2. Hypokalemia—treat <3.4 mEq/L

   a. Delay administration of any diuretic.

   b. Give 20 meq KCL over 1 hour (central line preferred) as:

      1. Serum K <3.4 mEq/L—2 doses

      2. Serum K <3.1 mEq/L—3 doses

      3. Serum K <2.9 mEq/L—4 doses

   a. If K remains >2.9 – <3.8 mEq/L—repeat above

   b. If K remains <3.2 mEq/L thereafter, consult MD (care to ensure >20 mcg/L of potassium infusion to prevent arrhythmia related death.

C. **Chloride (Cl)**—not independently treated

D. **Bicarbonate (HCO₃)**—not independently treated

E. **Magnesium (Mg)**

1. Hypermagnesemia—not independently treated
2. Hypomagnesemia—treat Mg <1.5 mg/dl
   a. Administer 4 gm magnesium sulfate ($MgSO_4$) over 2 hours repeat as indicated by subsequent laboratory assessment to maintain above goal levels.
   b. If Mg remains <1.5 mg/dl after 8 gm $MgSO_4$, consult MD.

F. **Phosphorus (P)**

1. Hyperphosphatemia—not independently treated
2. Hypophosphatemia—treat serum P <2.2 mg/dl (0.71 mmol/L)
   a. Give 30 mmol potassium or sodium phosphate over 3 hours and repeat (total 2 doses).
   b. If P remains <2.2 mg/dl (0.71 mmol/L) after 60 mmol sodium or potassium phosphate given, consult MD.

G. **Calcium (Ca)—Note:** Measure and treat only the ionized calcium value

1. Hyperionized calcemia—not separately treated. Withhold additional calcium.
2. Hypoionized calcemia—treat <4.4 mg/dl or <2.1 mEq/L or <1.1 mmol/L
   a. Give 10 cc 10% solution of calcium gluconate slow IV push
   b. Remeasure ionized Ca in 1 hour
   c. Repeat if ionized Ca is low
   d. If the ionized Ca remains low after 20 cc, 10% calcium gluconate is given, consult MD.

Guideline—Polyuria

Introduction

Polyuria may quickly lead to hypovolemia and hypoperfusion of donor organs. The causes of polyuria may be: (1) physiological diuresis after prior fluid administration. (2) Osmotic diuresis due to previous mannitol therapy or continuing hyperglycemia. (3) Diuresis from prescribed diuretics. (4) Diabetes insipidus. Physiological diuresis does not lead to hypotension, but all other forms may. If the donor demonstrates hypotension and polyuria, continue in this guideline, but refer also to Guideline—Hypotension. The urine output goal is 75–150 cc/hour.

Initial Assessment

A. Evaluate blood sugar per laboratory or finger stick measurement. Glucose values >200 mg/dl may contribute to polyuria. Refer to Guideline—Glucose management.
B. Stop any prescribed diuretic therapy
C. Calculate recent fluid intake/output balance and adjust intake to be 100 ml/hour less than total output. Example: You observe urine output over the last 3 hours averaged about 400 ml/hr. Adjust total IV fluid intake to equal about 300 ml/hr.
D. Follow q2 hr measurements of serum Na and glucose
F. If Na>148 mEq/L—assume excessive free H_2O loss has occurred, and proceed with treatment plan below.
G. If serum Na 135–147 mEq/L when last measured, observe urine output and repeated serum Na measurements. Maintain fluid intake 100 ml less than urine output each hour.

Treatment

A. Stop excessive intake (maintain intake 100 cc less than output until intake and ouput are equal and then maintain intake = output).
B. If urine output >250 cc above IV intake for the last 2 hours and serum Na>145 mEq/L when last measured, give 1 microgram desmopression (DDAVP) IV.
C. Begin replacement of urine output each hour cc/cc with 0.2% saline (no dextrose).
D. If urine output has not declined below 200 ml above intake (urine output >200 ml above fluid intake) in the

next 1 hour, give an additional 1 microgram of DDAVP intravenously.

E. If urine output has not decreased to <200 cc above IV intake (urine output >200 ml above fluid intake) and Na has not fallen to <146 Eq/L in 2 additional hours—consult MD.

Guideline—Acid–Base Treatment

Introduction

During donor care monitoring and treating the arterial pH becomes the primary acid–base goal. Because there are a few primary effects of hypocarbia or hypercarbia, the $PaCO_2$ will be adjusted to normalize the arterial pH (pH 7.35–7.45). Modifications of the mechanical ventilator to alter the PCO_2, and hence pH, are reviewed in the Guideline—Mechanical Ventilation.

Assessment

Because hospitals may report either the base Excess (BE) or base deficit (BD) with ABG results, both are included here.

A. **Acidosis:** Review the arterial blood gas (ABG) measurement obtained prior to manipulation of the mechanical ventilator recommended in the Rx Guideline—Mechanical Ventilation. Assess the BE or BD provided as part of the ABG results. IF the BE is more negative (–) than – 6 or the BD is more positive (+) than +6, metabolic acidosis is likely present.

B. **Alkalosis:** Review the ABG prior to adjustment of the mechanical ventilator as above. If the BE is more positive (+) than +6 or BD is more negative (–) than –6, metabolic alkalosis likely present, although very unusual during donor care.

Treatment

A. **Metabolic Acidosis:** If the arterial pH remains <7.32 after the changes recommended in the Rx Guideline—Mechanical Ventilation (Section IV A), administer one pre-mixed syringe (44 or 50 meq) $NaHCO_3$ slow IV push.

However, if the Na is concurrently >150 mEq/L, consult MD before giving $NaCO_3$. If the arterial pH remains <7.32 thereafter, consult MD.

B. **Metabolic Alkalosis:** If the arterial pH remains >7.45 after the changes recommended in the Mechanical Ventilation, consult MD.

Donor care flow sheet

Initial problem list   New problems

DATE

TIME										
Vital Signs										
Bld press S/D										
MAP										
Temp										
Heart rate										
Urine output										
ABG pH										
$PaCO_2$										
PaO_2										
HCO_3										
Chem Na										
K										
Cl										
Mg										
Ca										
Phos										
Glu										
other										
Hem HCT										
WBC										
Plts										
Coag PT										
PTT										
Fibrinogen										
Meds: Dopa										
µg/kg/min										
Norepi										
DDAVP (mcg)										
Other										
Fluids : 9% NS										
5% Alb										
Other										

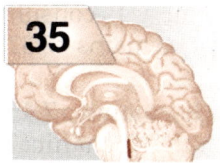

35
Is Brain Death Really Death? Is there any Degree of Uncertainty in its Diagnosis?

Well, the above questions are not entirely a new phenomenon: Doubts about what the science of death are and about the ability of the physicians to make the correct diagnosis of death have always existed. During the 19th century these controversies weakened, in parallel with the medical progresses (the invention of diagnostic tools as the stethoscope is a case in point), but during the last decades of the same century new controversies and doubts grew up resulting in a new wave of panic. Here too the scientific advances were instrumental: The possibility to keep the organs alive in the laboratory outside the organism and later possibility to culture and tissues *in vitro* and to transplant organs from an organism to another blurred the boundaries of death. There is a deep disagreement where brain death is synonymus with death. Death of the brain is not like the death in the traditional sense.

There are several proponents and opponents for the brain death criteria.

PROPONENTS VIEW

i. The President's Commission in its comments on the concepts of death have argued that the patients who suffered whole brain death should be viewed as dead.

   The primary reason was that (brain) and in particular the brain stem was the integrator of all the body organ systems. Without the integration, the commission reasoned that, continued functioning of the patients major organs systems in the ICU did not constitute that the organism lives.

ii. Once the diagnosis of brain death has been made the prognosis was certain that the patient would never regain consciousness and would develop asystole within a short time, despite continued aggressive intervention. The diagnostic certainty and uniformly dismal cardiac prognosis for brain death patients facilitated the acceptances of policies aimed at treatment withdrawal and organ retrival.

iii. One author points out the cost effectiveness equation as one reason why it is bad to ventilate corpse.

iv. Can an affluent society squander its resources in the preservation of intellectual life in the body of brain death?

v. The expense resuscitative efforts in terms of money, profession, personal and hospital facilities made it imperative that their unnecessary use be eliminated.

OPPONENTS VIEW

i. The death of a tissue in the brain death debate is not an impressing reality, but social category "social death". It is a question of which bodies are comfortable giving medicine or food as if they were alive.

ii. Would you trust a doctor who regards your body as an organism in need of healing but as a container of biologically useful materials.

iii. Although organ donors are declared dead they hardly resemble patients who have died from cardiopulmonary arrest. Infact they remind us in many ways of living patients. They are warm and retain a healthy color which is no surprise because their hearts continue to pump oxygenated blood through their body. Digestion, metabolism and elimination continue.

iv. To say a patient with a beating heart, a normal pulse, a normal blood pressure, a normal colour, and normal temperature is false.

v. While brain death criteria call for irreversible cessation of all brain functions, many persons who are declared brain dead retain significant brain functions such as production of arginine vasopressin.

vi. The fact is patient is dying and not dead.

vii. Determined to be dead but treated as alive.

viii. Some are not opposed to organ transplantation but very much are opposed to removing a vital organ from someone who if he/she is not yet dead, he/she will definitely be dead after the organ has been removed. This amounts to killing a patient.

ix. According to one Collaborative Study, 8% of those declared dead on the basis of those criteria omitting the EEG, still have cortical activity when evaluated by non-clinical means (EEG). Thus, action such as excision of a beating heart results in killing at least one in twelve under such circumstances.

x. A human being belongs to the species of *Homo sapiens* and, as such, is a person throughout his entire life, still when dying. There are attributes of a living human being that do not belong to other species, for example, thinking, judging, loving and acting. When it is predicted that a particular living human being will not be capable of demonstrating these attributes again, this living human being does then belong to other species. He is still a living human being, a living person. To say that a patient on a ventilator, declared "brain dead", is certain to die and is, therefore, no longer a person, is to deny reality.

xi. Great care must be taken not to declare a person dead even one moment before death has actually occurred. Death should only be declared after, not before, the fact as to declare prematurely is to commit a fundamental injustice. A person who is dying is still alive even a moment before death, and must be treated as much.

xii. Death ought not to be declared unless and until there is destruction of the entire brain, and of the respiratory and circulatory systems as well.

We strongly feel that once after having diagnosed brain death, then chances of survival of the other organs is negligible. Therefore at that particular time if the question arises regarding organ transplantation, one should duly consider it after prior consultation with the relations, because, by donating an organ the dead person is offering life to another individual.

With all the great respect for those who do not want to become organ donors. We for our part think that it is one of the most beautiful gifts one can give at the end of one's life, and that is a better life or even life to another human being.

Annexures

Annexure I

FORM-8

[See rule a(3)(a)and (b) of the THO Rules 1995]

We, the following members of the Board of medical experts after careful personal examination, hereby certify that

Shri/smt./km ....

Aged about ....

s/o, d/o, w/o, Shri ....

Resident of ....

.... is dead on account of permanent and irreversible cessation of all functions of the brain stem. The tests carried out by us and the findings therein are recorded in the brain stem death certificate annexed hereto.

Dated ....   Signature ....

1. R.M.P., Incharge of the Hospital in which brain stem death has occurred
2. R.M.P., nominated from the panel of names approved by the appropriate authority
3. Neurologist/Neuro-surgeon nominated from the panel of names approved by the appropriate authority
4. R.M.P., treating the aforesaid deceased person

BRAIN STEM DEATH CERTIFICATE

Patient Details:

1. Name of the patient   Shri/smt/km. ....

....

SO/DO/WO   Shri . ...

....

Sex .... Age ....

110

2. Home address ....
....
....

3. Hospital number ....

4. Name and address of next of ....

   kin or person responsible for the ....

   patient (if none exists, this must ....

   be specified) ....
   ....
   ....

5. Has the patient or next of kin ....

   agreed to any transplant? ....
   ....

6. Is this a police case? Yes.................... No ....

Pre-conditions

1. Diagnosis: Did the patient suffer from any illness or accident that led to irreversible brain damage? Specify details

....

....

....

Date and time of accident/onset of illness ....

Date and onset of non-responsive coma ....

2. Findings of board of medical experts:

   i. The following reversible causes of coma have been excluded: Intoxication (alcohol)

      Depressant drugs

      Relaxants (neuromuscular blocking agents)

	First Medical Examination		Second Medical Examination	
	1st	2nd	1st	2nd

Primary hypothermia

Hypovolemic shock

Metabolic or

endocrine disorders

Tests for absence of

brain stem functions

ii. Coma

iii. Cessation of spontaneous breathing

iv. Papillary size

v. Pupillary light reflexes

iv. Doll's head eye movements

vii. Corneal reflexes (both sizes)

viii. Motor response in any cranial nerve distribution, any responses to stimulation of face, limb or trunk

ix. Gag reflex

x. Cough (tracheal)

xi. Eye movements on coloric testing bilaterally

xii. Apnea tests as specified

xiii. Were any respiratory movements seen?

…...........................…………………………………………………………………………………

Date and time of first testing :

…...........................………………………………………………………………………………

This is to certify that the patient has been carefully examined twice after an interval of about six hours and on the basis of findings recorded above.

Shri/smt/km. ………………………………… Is declared brain stem dead

1. Medical Administrator incharge   2. Authorised specialist
   of the hospital
3. Neurologist/Neuro-surgeon   4. Medical Officer treating the patient

NB. I. The minimum time interval between the first testing and second testing will be six hours.

II. No. 2 and No. 3 will be co-opted by the administrator incharge of the hospital from the panel of experts approved by the appropriate authority.

Annexure II

Guidelines for apnea tests:

Patient should have a temperature of more than 35° centigrade euvolemic and with systolic pressure $=/>90$ mm of Hg.

i. The first apnea test should be performed only after 4 hours of coma associated with absence of brain stem reflexes. In the case of anoxic brain damage, this period should be extended to 12 hours.

ii. The physician involved in certifying brain death shall be present during ventilator removal to attest the presence of apnea if found.

iii. Ventilator manipulation is performed to raise the $PaCO_2=/>40$ mmHg.

iv. The patient should be hyperoxygenated with 100% oxygen for 15 minutes, while still on the ventilator, prior to the apnea test.

v. Either a blood gas or trending of $ETCO_2$ should be used to determine the adequacy of the baseline prior to the test. SPO_2 should be monitored during apnea test.

vi. Place the patient on 100% oxygenthrough a tracheal catheter with the tip towards the end of the tube with a continuous 6 L/min O_2 flow.

vii. The patient is taken off the ventilator in the presence of the physician certifying brain death. The patient is kept off the ventilator for a variable period of time (usually 3 to 8 minutes) to allow the $PaCO_2$ to rise $=/>55$ mmHg or $=/>15$ mmHg over baseline. During this time the patient is observed for respiratory movements.

viii. Test interpretations

    a. Positive test—implying apnea despite adequate stimulation

        i. Patient remains apneic, without respiratory movements

        ii. $PaCO_2$ is $=/>55$ mmHg or $=/>15$ mmHg from baseline

    b. Negative test—implying apnea is not present

      i. Respiratory efforts noted at any time during the test

    c. Indeterminate test

      i. $PaCO_2$ <55 mmHg or there is less than 15 mmHg increase over baseline.

    d. Indeterminate tests can either be repeated or another confirmatory test utilized.

ix. Apnea test should be aborted if the patient develops hypotension, or significant cardiac arrhythmias.

x. These norms will vary for patients less than 12 years and patients with major chest trauma.

Bibliography

1. Abbott SW. Death certification. In a Reference Handbook of the Medical Sciences, Vol III. New York: Wood, 1901.
2. Abdel-Dayem HM, Bahar RH, Sigurdsson GH, et al. The hollow skull: a sign of brain death in Tc-99m Hm-PAO brain scintigraphy. Clin Nuci Med 1989; 14:912–916.
3. Agich GJ. Jones, RP. Personal identity and brain death: a critical response. Philos Public Affairs 1985; 10:387–395.
4. Agich GJ, Jones, RP, Personal Identity and brain death: a critical response. Philos Public Affairs 1986; 15:267–274.
5. Aichner F, Felber S, Birbamer G, Luz G, Judmaler W, Schmutzhard E: Magnetic resonance: a noninvasive approach to metabolism, circulation, and morphology in human brain death. Ann Neurol 32:507–511, 1992.
6. Akabayashi A, Morioka M. Ethical issues raised by medical use of brain-dead bodies in the 1990's BioLaw 1991; 11:S531–S538.
7. Alderete JF, Jeri FR, Richardson EP Jr, et al. Irreversible coma: a clinical electroencephalographic and neuropathological study. Trans Am Neurol Assoc 32:507–511, 1992.
8. Allegheny County Ad Hoc Committee on Tissue Transplantation. Protocol for the determination of death. Penn Med 1969; 72(3):17–20.
9. Allen, N: Life or death of the brain or cardiac arrest. Neurology 27:805/806, 1977.
10. American Electroencephalographic Society. Guidelines in EEG, Willoughby, OH: American electroencephalographic Society, 1976.
11. American Neurological Association: Revised statement regarding methods of determining that the brain is dead. Trans. Am. Neurol. Assoc. 102:192–193, 1977.
12. An appraisal of the criteria of cerebral death; a summary statement. A collaborative study, JAMA 1976; 237:982–986.
13. Anonymuos, Anencephalic of the infants as sources of transplantable organs. Hastings Cent Rep 1988; 18:28–30.
14. Aries P. Western Attitudes toward Death; From the Middle Ages to the Present, Ranum P (transl). Baltimore: Johns Hopkins, 1974.

15. Aries P. The Hour of Our Death, New York; Knopf, 1981.

16. Arnold H, Ansorg P, Voigtsberger P, et al. Beitrag der Pulsationsechoenzephalographer zur Todeszeitbestimmung. Acta Neurochir (Wien) 1972: 27:263–275.

17. Arras JD, Shinnar S. Anencephalic newbords as organ donors: a critique, JAMA 1988; 259:2284–2285.

18. Artru F, Terrier A, Gibert I, Messaoudi K, Charlot M, Naous H, Jourdan C. Technical aspects and clinical reliability of intracranial pressure monitoring with a parenchymal fiberoptic transducer. Ann Fr Anesth Reanim 11:424–429, 1992.

19. Ashwal S, Schneider S. Failure of electroencephalography to diagnose brain death in comatose children. Ann Neurol 1979; 6:512–517.

20. Ashwal S, Schneider S. Thompson J. Xenon computed tomography measuring cerebral blood flow in the determinaton of brain death in children. Ann Neurol 1989, 25:539–546.

21. Ashwal S, Smith, AJK, Torres F, et al. Radionuclide bolus angiography; a technique for verification of brain death in infants and children. J Pediatr 1977; 91:772.

22. Baird PA, Sadovnick AD. Survival in infants with anencephaly Clin Pediatr 1984; 23:268–271.

23. Barton HM. Cruzan v Missouri; will the real meaning please stand up? Texas Med 1990; 86:18–19.

24. Becker, DP, Robert, CM, Jr., Nelson, JR, and Stern, WE: An evaluation of cerebral death, Neurology 20:459–462, 1970.

25. Beecher, HK. A definition of irreversible coma: report of the Ad Hoc Committee of the Harvard Medical School to Examine the definition of Brain Death. JAMA 1968; 205:337–340.

26. Beecher, HK: After the "Definition of irreversible coma". N.Engl. J.Med.281:1070–1071, 1969.

27. Beller FK, Reeve J. Brain life and brain death: the anencephalic as an explanatory example: a contribution to transplantation J Med Philos 1989; 15:5–23.

28. Bendann E. Death Customs: An Analytical Study of Burial Rites, 1st ed, reprinted. London: Dawson, 1969.

29. Bennett, D.R., Hughes, J.R., Korein, J et al: Atlas of the Electroencephalography in Coma and Cerebral Death, EEG at the Bed side or in the Intensive Care Unit, Raven Press, New York, 1976.

30. Benzel EC, Gross CD, Hadden TC, et al. The apnea test for the determination of the brain death. J Neurosurg 1989; 71:191–194.

31. Berkutov AN, Tsybulyak GN, Pashkovsky EV, et al. Prognosis of severe trauma and diagnosis of brain death in the donor after extraction of the heart for grafting. Eksp Khir Anesteziol 1969; 2:29–34.

32. Bichat X. Physiological Reasearches upon Life and Death, 2nd French ed, Walkins T (transl). Philadelphia: Smith and Maxwell, 1809.

33. Black P Mcl. Brain death: Parts 1 and 2, N Engl J Med 1978; 299:338–344, 393–401.

34. Black P Mcl. Conceptual and practical issues in the declaration of death by brain criteria. Neurosurg Clin North Am 1991; 2:493–501.

35. Black, PM: Brain Death. N.Engl J.Med. 299:338–344, 393–401, 1978.

36. Brante T. Hallberg M. Brain or heart? The controversy over the concept of death. Social stud science 1991: 2:389–413.

37. Brieley, JB, Adams JH, Graham, DI, et al: Neocortical death after cardiac arrest. Lancet 2:560–565, 1971.

38. Brody B. The essence of humanity in the abortion and the sanctity of human life: a philosophical view. Hastings Cent Rep 1972; 2:187–189.

39. Brouardel P. Death and Sudden Death, 2nd ed. New York: William Wood, 1902.

40. Buchner H, Schuchart V, Reliability of electroencephalogram in the diagnosis of brain death. Eur Neurol 1990: 30:138–141.

41. Byme PA, O'Reilly S, Quay PM, Brain Death—an opposing view point. JAMA 1979:242:1985–1990.

42. Campbell J, the Masks of God, Primitive Mythology, New York Viking, 1954.

43. Canadian Medical Association Statement on death, November 1968. Can Med Assoc J 1968; 99:1266–1267.

44. Capron, Am. Anencephalic donors: separate the dead from the dying, Hastings Cent Rep 1987; n17:5, 9.44. Capron, AM. Criteria of death. J Med Ethics 1990; 16:167 (letter).

45. Cefalo RC, Engelhardt HT Jr. The use fetal and anencephalic tissue for transplantation J.Med Philos 1989; 14:25–43.

46. Chatrian, GE: Electrophysiological evaluation of brain death: A critical appraisal. In Aminoff, M.J.(ed): Electrodiagnosis in Clinical Neurology, Churchill-Livingstone, New York, Edinburg, London 1980.

47. Chippa, KH Choi. S, and Young, RR. Short latency somato-sensory evoked potentials following median nerve stimulation

in patients with neurological lesions. Prog. Clin Neurophysiol. 7:264–281, 1980.

48. Conference of Medical Royal Colleges: Diagnosis of brain death. Br.Med J 2:1187–1188, 1976.

49. Conference of Royal Colleges and Faculties of the United Kingdom: Diagnosis of brain death. Lancet 2:1069–1070, 1976.

50. Counsell national de l; Orbre des Medecins. Le prplement d' unorgane sur in "Mort EN SURVIE ARTIFICELLES." Presse Med 1968; 74:952.

51. Council for International Organisation of Medical Sciences (CIOMS). Sur la greffe du Coeur. Presse Med 1968; 76:390.

52. Crafoord CC. Cerebral death and transplantations era. Chest 1969; 55:141–145.

53. Cranford RE. Brain death: concept and criteria. Minn Med 1978; 61:561–563.

54. Cullen, DJ. Results and costs of intensive care. Anesthesiology 47:203–216, 1977.

55. Cushing H. Some experimental and clinical observations concerning states of increased intracranial tension. Am J Med Sci 1902; 124:375–400.

56. Cushman R, Holm S. Death, democracy and public ethical choice. Bioethics 1990; 4:237–252.

57. Darby J, Yonas H, Brenner RP. Brain stem death with persistent EEG activity, evaluation by xenon-enhanced computer tomography. Crit Care Med 1987; 15:519–521.

58. Darby JM, Yonas H, Gur D, et al. Xenon-enchanced computer tomography in brain death, Arch Neurol 1987; 44:551–554.

59. Darby JM, Stein K, Grenwik AM, Peacock WJ, et al. Approach to Management of the Heartbeating "Brain Death" Organ Donor. JAMA 261:2222–8, 1989.

60. Defining Death: A Report in the Legal and Ethical issues in the Determination of Death. Washington DC: President's Commission for the Study of Ethical Problems in Medicine and Bio-Medical and Behavioural Research, 1981.

61. Definition of the signs and time of death. Statement by the Commission no Reanimation and Organ Transplantation appointed by the German Society of Surgery. Ger Med Mon 1968; 13:359.

62. De la Riva A Gonzalez FM, Liamas-Elvira JM, et al. Diagnosis of brain death superiority of perfusion studies with 99mTc HMPAO over conventional radiouclide cerebral angiography. Br J Radiol 1992; 65:289–294.

63. Determination of Death, 2nd ed; and Minority Report. The New York State Task Force on Life and the Law, 1989.

64. Deutsh E. The use of human tissue, particularly foetal tissue, in neurosurgery. Med Law 1990; 9:671–674.

65. Diagnosis of brain death. Lancet 1976; 2:1096–1070.

66. Dictionnaire des Sciences Medicales en Soxiante Tomes. Paris CLF Panckoucke, 1818.

67. Drake B, Ashwal S, Schneider S: Determination of cerebral death in the pediatric intensive care unit. Pediatrics 78:107–112, 1986.

68. Eelco F.M. Wijdicks, Panayiotis N. Varelas, Gray S. Gronseth and David M. Greer, Neurology 2010; 74; 1911–1918.

69. Fakler Rogers MC, Is brain really cessation of all intracranial function? J Pediatr 1987; 110:84–86.

70. Faldman EA, Defining death: organ transplants, traditional and technology in Japan. Soc Sci Med 1988; 27:339–343.

71. Flanagan, RJ, Prior, JG, Raper SM, Widdop. B, and Volans G.N., Letter to editor. Lancet 1:283, 1981–68.

72. Fletcher JC Anderson WF, Germ-line gene theraphy—a new stage of debate. Law Med Health Care 1992; 20:26–39.

73. Florida Statue. Ann 1990 (West) Sec 82.085 (2).

74. Fost N, Organs from anencephalic infants: an idea whose time has not yet come. Hastings Cent Rep 1988; 18:5–10.

75. Francisaco CJ, III. Organ donation and transplantation—what every physician should Texas Med 1988; 84:92–95.

76. Freeman JM, Ferry PC: New brain death guidelines in children: further confusion. Pediatrics 81:301–303, 1988.

77. French JM, Modes of death. In a Reference Handbook of Medical Sciences, Vol III. New York: Wood, 1901.

78. Galaske RG, Schober O, Heyer R, 99mTc-HM-PAO and 123/-amphetamine cerebral acintigraphy—a new, noninvasive method of determination of brain death in children. Eur J Nucl Med 1988; 14:446–452.

79. Ganes T, Lunder T, EEG and evoked potentials in comatose patients with severe brain damage. Electroencephalogr Clin Neurophysiol 1988; 69:6–13.

80. Garry DJ, Caplan AL, Vawter DE, et al. Are there really alternatives to the use fetal tissue from elective abortion in transplantation research? N Engl J Med 1992; 327:1592–1595.

81. George MS, Establishing brain death the potential role of nuclear medicine in the search for a reliable confirmatory test. Eur J Nucl Med 1992; 18:75–77.

82. Gilgamesh. Leonard WL (trans). Avon, CT: The Limited Editions Club, 1974.

83. Goldie, WD, Chippa, KH, and Young, RR Brain stem auditory evoked responses in brain death. Neurology 31:248–256, 1981.

84. Goodman, JM, Mishkin, FS, and Dyken, M: Determination of brain death by isotope angiography. JAMA. 209:1869–1872, 1969.

85. Greem MB, Wikler D, Brain death and perconnel identity. Philos Public Affairs 1980; 9:105–133.

86. Greenberg MS: Brain Death, in Green MS (ed): Handbook of Neurosurgery, Lakeland FL, Greenberg Graphics, 1994, pp. 120–126.

87. Grigg MM<Kelly MA, Celesia GG, et al. Electroencephalographic activity after brain death. Arch Neurol 1987; 44:948–954.

88. Guidelines for the determination of death. Report of the medical consultants on diagnosis of death to the President's commission for the Study of Ethical Problems in Medicine and Biochemical and Behavioral Research. JAMA 1981: 246:2184–2186.

89. Gurvitch, AM: Determination of the death and reversibility of post anoxic coma in animals. Resuscitation 3:1–26, 1974.

90. Habenstein RW lamers WM. Funeral Customs the World Over. Milwauke, WI: Bulfin Printers, 1960.

91. Hall JW III, Mackey—Hargadine JR, Kim EE. Auditory brain stem responses in determination of brain death. Arch Otolaryngol 1985; 111:613–620.

92. Hall JW III, Tucker DA, Sensory evoked responses in the intensive care unit. Ear Hear 1986; 7:220–232.

93. Hamlin H. Life on death of EEG. JAMA 1964; 190:112–114.

94. Hardy RC. Updated definition of brain death in Texas. Texas Med 1991; 87:76–81.

95. Harrison JE. Prolegomena to the Study of Greek Religion. London: Merlin Press 1961.

96. Hassler W, Steinmetz H, Pirschel J: Transcranial Doppler study of intracranial circulatory arrest. J Neurosurg 71:195–201, 1989.

97. Hawaii, Hawaii Rev Sat 327 C-1, Supp 1984.

98. Heytens L, Verlooy J, Gheuens J, et al. Lazarus Sign and Extensor Posturing in A Braib-Death Patient. J Neurosurg 71:449–51, 1989.

99. Hiatt, HH: "Protectin the medical commons: who is responsible? N Engl J. Med 293:235–241, 1975.

100. Hopkins JP, New laws on patient treatment decisions. Texas Med 1989; 85:54–57.

101. Hughes JR. Limitations of the EEG in coma and brain death. Ann NY Acadd Sci 1978; 315:121–136.
102. Lcard S. Du danger de la mort apparenete. Presse Med 1904; 12:521–525.
103. Infant with anencephaly. N Engl J Med 1990; 322:669–674.
104. Ingvar DH, Widen L. Hjamdod-Sammanfattningav ett symposium, Lakartidningen 1972; 69:3804–3814.
105. Ivan LP. Irreversible brain damage and related problems: pronouncement of death. L Am Geriatr Soc 1970; 18:816–822.
106. Ivan LP: Spinal Reflexes in Cerebral Death, Neurology 23:650–2, 1973.
107. Iyer TKK. Kidneys for transplant—"opting Out" law in Singapore. Forensic Sci Int 1987; 35:131–140.
108. Jahrig K. Grenzen der Lebenserhaltung beim Neugeborenen. Zur Bestimmug des Himtodes in den Neoatalzeit. Kinderarztl Prax 1979; 47:65–70.
109. Jensen-Juul, P: Criteria of Brain Death, Selection of Donors for Transplantation, Munksgaard, Copenhagen, 1970.
110. Jennett, B. Gleave, J., and Wilson P. Brain death in three neurosurgical units. Br. Med. J. 282:533–539, 1981.
111. Jorgenson, EO: Spinal man after brain death. Acta Neurochir, 28:259–273, 1973.
112. Jorgenson, EO: Brain death, Retrospective survey. Lancet 1:378–3799, 1981.
113. Jorgenson, EO., and Mallchow-Moller, A: Cerebral Prognostic signs during cardiopulmonary resuscitation. Resuscitation 6:217–225, 1978.
114. Kalish RA (ed): Death and Dying: Views from Many Cultures. Farmingdale, MY: Baywood Publ 1980.
115. Kassirer JP, Angell M. The use of fetal tissue in research in Parkinson's disease. N Engl J Med 1992; 327:1591–1592.
116. Kaste. M, Hollborn, M, and Palo. J. Diagnosis and management of brain death. Br. Med J 1; 525–527, 1979.
117. Kaufer C, Penin H, Dux A et al. Zerebraler Zirulationsstillstand bir hirntod durch Hypoxidosen. Forsch Med 1969; 87:713–717.
118. Kautman HH, Geister FH, Kopitnik T, et al. Detection of brain death in barbiturate coma: the dilemma of an intracranial pulse. Neurosurgery 1989; 25:275–278.
119. Kearney W, Vawter DE, Gervals KG. Fetal tissue research and the misread compromise. Hasting Cent Rep 1991; 21:712.
120. Kimura R. Anencephalic organ donation: a Japanese case. J Med Philos 1989; 14:97–102.

121. Kimura R, Japan's dilemma with the definition of death. Kennedy Inst Ethics J 1991; 1:123–131.

122. Kirkland LL. Family Refusal to accept brain death and termination of life support: to whom is the physician responsible? J Clin Ethics 1991:2:171.

123. Kohrman MH, Spivack BS. Brain death infants: sensitivity and specificity of current criteria. Pediatr Neurol 1990: 6:47–50.

124. Korein J. (ED): Brain Death: Interrelated medical and social issues. Ann N.Y. Acad. Sci. 315:1–454, 1978.

125. Korein, J, Braunstein, P, George, A, et al: Brain Death: 1. Angiographic correlation with the radioisotopic bolus technique for evaluation of critical deficit of cerebral flow. Ann. Neurol 2: 195–205, 1977.

126. Kosteljanetz M, Ohrstrom JK, Skjodt S, et al. Clinical brain death with preserved arterial circulation. Acta Neurol Scand 1988; 78:418–421.

127. Kramer W, Tuynman JA, Acute intracranial hypertension—an experimental investigation, Brain Res 1967; 6:686–705.

128. Laurin, NR, Driedger AA, Hurwitz GA, et al. Cerebral perfusion imaging with technetium 99m HM-PAO in brain death and severe central nervous system injury. J Nucl Med 1989; 30:1627–1635.

129. Levin SD, Whyte RK; Brain death sans frontiers. N Engl J Med 318:852–853, 1988.

130. Levy, DE, Bates, D, Caronna, JJ, et al. Prognosis in non-traumatic coma. Ann. Intern. Mede. 94:293–301, 1981.

131. Lock M. Reaching consensus about death; heart transplantation and cultural identity in Japan. Society 1989; 13:15–26.

132. Lorenz R. Kriterien der Himtatigkeit in lebensbedrohenen Zustanden—ein Beitrag zur Frage des zentralen todes. Acta Neurochir (Wien) 1969; 20:309–329.

133. Lucas, BA, Pitts Lh, Ketter CS et al. The neurosurgeon's role in organ procurement. Am Assoc Neurol Surg Bull Winter, 1992; 36:40–47.

134. Lynch J, Eldadah MK, Brain—death criteria currently used by pediatric intensivitis, Clin Pediatr 1992; 31:14–24.

135. Mandel S, Arenas A Scasta D; Spinal automatism in cerebral death. N Engl J Med 307:501, 1982.

136. Marks SJ, Zisfein J: Apneic oxygenation in apnea tests for brain death. A control trial Arch Neurol 47:1066–1068, 1990.

137. Marshall TD. Canadian regulation of the medical use fetal tissue in research and therapy. Can Med Assoc J 1989; 140:1021–1022.

138. Marshall TK. Premature burial. Med Leg J 1967; 35:14–24.
139. May WF, Religious obstacles and warrents for the donation of body parts. Transplant Proc 1988; 20 (1 Supp 1): 1079–1083.
140. Mc Gillivray BC. Anencephaly: the potential for survival. Transplant Proc 1988; 20(4 Suppl 5); 9–16.
141. Meister SH, Trachtman, H. Parental attitudes toward organ transplantation. Pediatr. Nephrol 1989; 3:86–88.
142. Mohandas. A. Chou SN. Brain death. A clinical and pathological study. J Neurosurg 1971; 35:211–218.
143. Mollaret P, Betrand I, Mollaret H, Coma depasse et necroses nerveuses centrals massives. Rev Neurol (Paris) 1959; 101:116–139.
144. Mollaret P, Goulon M, Le coma depasse: (Memoire preliminaire), Rev Neurol (Paris) 1959; 101:3–15.
145. Molloy A. Attitudes to Medical Ethics among British Muslim Medical practitioners. L Med Ethics 1980; 6:139–144.
146. Molnar T, Fetus selection: the French perspective. Hum Life Rev 1984; 10:67–72.
147. Montgomery TM, cited by Tebb W, Vollum EP, Premature Burial and How it May Be Prevented. London: Swan Sonnenschein & Co. Ltd., 1905.
148. Morayati SJ, Nagle CE. The determination of death and changing role of medical imaging. Radiographics 1988; 8:967–979.
149. Netherlands Red Cross Society. Summary of the Report of the Ad Hoc Committee on Organ Transplantation, 1971.
150. New Jersey Advance Directives of Health Care and Declaration of Death Acts. State of New Jersey, November, 1991.
151. New Jersey Declaration of Death Act. P.L. 1991 Ch 90. Kennedy Inst Ethics J 1991; 1:289–292.
152. Nudeshmia J. Obstacles of brain death and organ transplantation in Japan. Lancet, 1991: 338:1063–1064.
153. Olick RS. Brain Death, religious freedom and public policy: New Jersy's landmark legislative initiative. Kennedy Inst Ethics J 1991; 1:275–288.
154. Oppenhiem H. Textbook of Nervous Diseases for physicians and students. Vol 2 Bruce A (trans). Edinburgh: Dorein Press, 1911.
155. Ota K. Present status of kidney donation in Japan. Transplant Proc 1991; 23:2512–2513.
156. Ouknine, G: Bedside procedures in the diagnosis of brain death. Resuscitation 4:159–177, 1975.

157. Outwater KM, Rockoff MA: Diabetes insipidus accompanying brain death in children. Neurology 34:1243–1246, 1984.

158. Pallis C. ABC of brain stem death: pitfalls and safeguards. Br Med J 1982; 285:1780.

159. Pallis, C. Prognostic value of brain stem lesion. Lancet 1:379, 1981.

160. Pasternak JF, Volpe JJ. Full recovery from prolonged brain stem failure following intraventricular haemorrhage. J. Pediatr 1979; 95:1046–1049.

161. Patel YP, Gupta SM, Baston R, et al. Brain Death: confirmation by radionuclide cerebral angiography. Clin Nucl Med 1988; 13:438–442.

162. Pernick MS, Back from the grave: recurring controversies over defining and diagnosing death in history. In Zaner rM (ed): Death Beyond Whole-Brain Criteria. Philosophy and Medicine Series, 31. Boston: Kluwer, 1988, pp 17–74.

163. Perry C, Schneider LK, Cryopreserved embryos: who shall decide their fate? J Leg Med 1992; 13:463–500.

164. Pistoia F, Johnson DW, Darby JM, et al. The role of xenon CT measurements of cerebral blood flow in the clinical determination of brain death, Am L Neuroradiol 1991; 12:97–103.

165. Powner, DJ, and Grenvik, A: Triage in patient care: from expected recovery in brain death. Heart and Lung 8:1103–1108, 1979.

166. Prior, P: Brain death, Lancet 1:1142, 1981.

167. President's Commission for the Study of Ethical Problems in Medicine: Guidelines for the Determination of Death. JAMA 246:2184–6, 1981.

168. Regional Organ Bank of Illinois, Chicago, IL.

169. Reid RH, Gulenchyn KY, Ballinger JR, Clinical use of Technetium 99m HM-PAO for determination of brain death. J Nucl Med 1989; 15:203–208.

170. Rispler-Chaim V. Islamic Medical Ethics in the 20th century. J Nucl Med Ethics 1990; 16:5–7.

171. Rix BA. Danish Ethics Council rejects brain death as criterion of death J Med Ethics 1990; 16:5–7.

172. Ropper AH. Unusual spontaneous movements in brain-dead patients. Neurology 1984; 34:1089–1092.

173. Ropper AH, Kennedy SK, Russell L. Apnea testing in the diagnosis of brain death: Clinical and physiological observations. J Neurosurg 1984; 34:1089–1092.

174. Rosner F. Definition of death in Jewish law. NY State J Med 1983; 83:973–978.

175. Rosner F. The traditionalist Jewish physician and modern biomedical ethics and problems. J Med Philos 1983; 8:225–241.

176. Rosner F, Risenberg HM, Bennett AG et al. The anencephalic fetus and new born as organ donors. NY State J Med 1988; 88:860–366.

177. Rosoff SD, Schwab RS. The EEG in establishing brain death: a 10-year report with criteria and legal safeguards in the 50 states. Electrocencephalogr Clin Neurophysiol 1969; 24:283–284.

178. Rothenbrg LS. The anencephalic neonate and brain death: an international review of medical ethical and legal issues. Transplant Proc 1990; 22: 1037–1039.

179. Royal Colleges and their faculties in the United Kingdom. Diagnosis of Brain Death. Br J med 1976; 2:1187–1188; Lancet 1976; 2:1069–1070.

180. Sachedina AA Islamic views on organ transplantation. Transplant Proc 1988; 20 (1 Supp 1): 1084–1088.

181. Sarma V. Medical ethics: Rules for fetal research adopted. Nature 1983; 306:308

182. Sass H-M. Brain life and Brain death: a proposal for a normative agreement. J Med philos 1989; 14: 45–59.

183. Sassower R, Grodin MA. Epidemiology questions concerning death. Death Stud 1986: 10:341–353.

184. Schafer, JA, and caronna. JJ, Duration of apnea needed to confirm brain death. Neurology, 28:661–668, 1978.

185. Schoen WL. Conflict in the parameters defining life and death in Missouri statues. Am J Law Med 1990; 16:555–580.

186. Schultze OH, Legal status of cadaver. In A reference of Hand book of the Medical Sciences, Vol II New York: Wood, 1901.

187. Schwab RS Potts F, Bonazzi A. EEG as an aid in determining death in the presence of cardiac activity (ethical, legal and medical aspects). Electroencephalogr Clin Neurophysiol 1963; 15:147–148 (abstr).

188. Shewmon DA. The probability of inevitability: inherent impossibility of validating criteria for brain death or "irreversibility" through clinical studies, Stat Med 1987; 6:535–553.

189. Silverman DA, Anencephaly: selected medical aspects. Hastings Cent Rep 1988; 18: 11–19.

190. Silverman D, Saunders MG, Schwab RS, et al. Irreversible coma associated with electrocerebral silence. Neurology 1970; 20:525–533.

191. Silverman D, Saunders MG, Schwab RS, et al. Cerebral death and the electroencephalographis Society on EEG Critaria for Determination of Cerebral Death. JAMA 1969; 209: 1505–1511.

192. Snelling LK, Helfaer MA, traystman RJ, et al. Comparison of cerebral blood flow by radionuclide cerebral angiography and by microspheres in cats. Crit care Med Bull 1970; 23:395–401.

193. Solnitsky O. Death of the brain: A vital diagnostic factor in organ transplantation. Georgetown Med Bull 1970; 23:94–103.

194. Sontag S. Illness as Metephor. New York: Farrar Straus & Giroux 1978.

195. Spann W. Vorstellungen zur Gestgebung liber den tatasachlichen Todeszeitpunkt. Munch Med Wochenschr 1969; 111; 2253–2255.

196. Starr. A; Auditory Brain stem responses in brain death. Brain 99:543–544, 1976.

197. Steinberg A. The definition of death in medicine anr Jewish law. In Rosner F (ed): Medicine and Jewish Law. Northvale, NJ. Aronson Inc, 1990.

198. Stockkard JJ, and Sharbrough, FW: Unique contributions of short-latency sensory evoked potentials to neurological diagnosis. Prog Clin. Neurophysiol. 7:231–236, 1980.

199. Takeuchi K, Takeshita H, Takakura K, et al. New Japanese criteria of brain death: Brain death Study Group. Neurosurg Rev. 1989: 12 (Suppl 1): 265–275.

200. Tan WS, Wilbur AC, Jaffar JJ, et al. Brain Death: use of Dynamic CT and intravenous digital subtraction angiography. Am J Neuroradiol 1987; 8:123–125.

201. Task Force for the Determination of Brain Death in Children. Guidelines for the Determination of Brain Death in Children. Arch Neurol 44; 587–8, 1987.

202. Task Force for the Determinations of Brain Death in Children: Guidelines for the Determination of Brain Death in Children. Arch Neurol 44; 587–8, 1987.

203. Texas Statue Dealing with Brain Death. Vemo's Texas code Annot. Title 8A Section 671 001.

204. Thompson JR, Ashwal S, Schneider S, et al. Comparison of cerebral blood flow measurements by xenon computed tomography and dynamic brain, scintigraphy in clinically brain dead children. Acta RADIOL 1986; Suppl 369:675–679.

205. Turmel A, Roux A, Bojanowski MW: Spinal man after declaration of brain death. Neurosurgery 28:298–302, 1991.

206. Tsuji KT. The Buddhist view if the body and organ transplantation. Transplant Proc 1988; 20:1076–1078, 192. Ueki K, Takeuchi K, Katsurada K, Clinical study of brain death, Presented at the Fifth International Congress of Neurological Surgery, Tokyo, 1973.

207. US Navy Department, Determination of cerebral death or electroencephalographic silence. Bumed Instruct 5306.24, April 15, 1954.

208. Valery P. La fausse morte. In Gide A (ed): Arthologie de la poesie Francaise. Paris: Bibl de la Pleiade, Gallimard, 1949.

209. Van Bunnen Y, Delcour C, Wery D, et al. Intravenoud digital subtraction angiography; criteria of brain death. Ann Radiol (Paris)1989; 32:279–281.

210. Vernant JP. The Origins of Greek Thought, Ithace, NY: Cornell University Press, 1982.

211. Virginnia Code 54a 325.7, 1982.

212. Walker AE. The death of brain. Johns Hopkins Med J 1969; 124:190–201.

213. Walker AE Cerebral Death. 2nd ed. Baltimore: Urban & Schwar zenberg, n1981.

214. Walters JW, Anencephalic organ procurement: should the law be changed? Biolaw 1987; 2(Suppl): 83–89.

215. Walters JW. Approaches to ethical decision making in the neonatal intensive care unit. Am J Dis Child 1988; 142:825–830.

216. Walters, JW. Anencephalic infants as organ sources. Bioethics 1991; 5:326–341,203. Walters JW. Proximate personhood as a standard for making difficult treatment decisions; imperiled newborns as a case study. Bioethics 1992; 6:12–22.

217. Walters LW, Ashwal S. Organ prolongation in anencephalic infants: ethical and medical issues. Hastings Cent rep 1988; 18;19–27.

218. Warwersik J. Kriterien des Todes uter dem Aspekt der reanimation. Chirurg 1968; 39:345–348.

219. Weiss DW. Organ transplantation: medical ethics and Jewish law. Transplant Proc 1988; 20 (Suppl 1): 1071–1072.

220. Wheeldon D. Thoracic organ preservation. Perfusion 1991; 6:191–202.

221. Willke JC, Andrusko D. Personhood redux. Hasting Cent Rep 1988: 18:30–33.

222. Winslow GR. Anencephalic infants as organ sources: should the law be changed? J Pediatr 1989; 115:825–832.

223. Winslow J. Dissertation sur l'Incertitude des signes de la morte at de l'abusd des Enterrements et Embaumements Preciptes. Transl from Latin with commentary by Jacques—Jean Bruhier d' Ablaincourt. Paris: Morel, 1740.

224. Withholding and withdrawing medical care—1986 update. Texas Med 1986; 82:67–70.

225. Working Party, Health Departments, Great Britain and Northern Ireland. The Removal of Cadaveric Organs for transplantation: A code of Practice, London: Stationery office, 1979.

226. Yamauchi M. Transplantation in Japan. Br Med J 1990; 301:507.

227. Yamauchi M. Waiting for Japanese transplants. Br Med J 1991; 303:266.

228. Yonemoto S. Ad Hoc research Committee on Brain Death and Organ transplantation. Social Sci Med 1991; 33:215.

229. Youmans JR, Keller TM, Alknse JR, Cerebral Death. In Youmans Jr(ed): Neurological Surgery, 2nd ed. Philadelphia: Saunders, 1982, pp. 746–761.

230. Ypunger Sj, Landefeld CS, Coulton CJ, et al. "Brain Death" and organ retrieval; A cross sectional survey of knowledge and concepts among health professionals. JAMA 1989; 261:2205–2210.

231. Zamer RM. Anencephalics as organ donors. J Med Philos 1989; 14:61–78.

232. The quality Standards Subcommittee of the American academy of Neurology. Practice parameters for determining brain death in adults (summary statement) Neurology 1995; 45:1012–4.

Index